Treatment of Aphasia

CLINICAL UPDATES IN SPEECH-LANGUAGE PATHOLOGY SERIES

Note from an Advisory Editor

The heart of speech-language-hearing pathology is clinical practice. For the most part, clinical practitioners have had to create clinical procedures out of the stuff of their own practice or from the hints contained in general books on each of the disorders. Until now. The *Clinical Updates Series* changes that. Each book in this series emphasizes daily clinical practice. The emphasis is on how to do evaluation and treatment. Of course, the books are cookbooks. They are not grocery lists, however, nor are they esoteric analyses of cultural differences about what is edible. Readers will find discussions of specific techniques and specific guidelines for selecting and ordering materials and procedures. These books are proof that good clinicians can be good writers. They are written with the knowledge that good clinicians are like good cooks—they use what they like and need, and they adapt and change as appropriate. And they always double the mushrooms.

Jay Rosenbek

Treatment of Aphasia
A Language-Oriented Approach

Cynthia M. Shewan, Ph.D.
Director, Research Division
American Speech-Language-Hearing Association

Department of Communicative Disorders
The University of Western Ontario
London, Ontario

Donna L. Bandur, M.Cl.Sc.
Speech Pathology Department
University Hospital
London, Ontario

 College-Hill Press, San Diego, California

College-Hill Press, Inc.
4284 41st Street
San Diego, California 92105

Library of Congress Cataloging in Publication Data
Main entry under title:

Shewan, Cynthia M.
    Treatment of aphasia.

    Bibliography: p.
    Includes index.
    1. Aphasia—Treatment. 2. Speech therapy.
I. Bandur, Donna L., 1951–   . II. Title.
[DNLM: 1. Aphasia—therapy.   2. Language Therapy—
methods. WL 340.5 S554t]
RC425.S5   1986   616.85'5206   86-2305

IBSN 0-88744-188-2

Printed in the United States of America

This book is dedicated to

Dr. Ronald Melzack, who kindled my inquisitiveness
Mrs. Laura Lee, who taught me about language
Dr. Gerald Canter, who made loving aphasia such a high probability event

Cynthia M. Shewan

CONTENTS

FOREWORD

Does it surprise you, the reader, to know that the Foreword to this language-modality focused work in treatment for aphasia has been written by an unreconstructed functionalist, whose own work in aphasia focuses on messages, communicative intents, and whatnot? Well, don't be so surprised. In this challenging world of clinical aphasiology, one can only cheer Cynthia Shewan and Donna Bandur, who have accomplished a functionalist's dream. In this volume they have stated unequivocally their rationale for the way they treat aphasic patients, then have presented a series of quite specific techniques that flow naturally from their rationale. They have also provided data to back up their work. A true functionalist cannot find fault with that, for it is truly the bottom line, a principled approach to treatment.

I am honored to be writing this Foreword. Aphasia rehabilitation needs specific, objective, and clearly articulated techniques for improving the aphasic condition. The opportunity to write these brief comments allows me in some small way to be a part of this very impressive effort. I have known and respected Dr. Shewan for some years. Her energy and her creative, problem-solving approach to thinking about aphasic patients are matched by her care and regard for them as people. I think these qualities shine through in these pages. I do not know Ms. Bandur, but because this is a collaborative work, it seems clear that she shares these qualities. One can only hope that Dr. Shewan and Ms. Bandur will continue to treat aphasic patients, whose lives they know how to influence positively. One can also hope that others who treat aphasic patients will study this book carefully. They will profit from it. There are literally hundreds of well-thought-out ideas here, and a promise of wide applicability.

I believe that this book might well portend a new area in clinical aphasiology. We are finally becoming self-confident enough to take chances and to risk sharing ideas specifically and directly with others, to put our beliefs about what works best in treatment out there for others to scrutinize, to challenge to use. We are beginning to put our clinical theories into very specific terms and into coherent frameworks. Our ideas are becoming more important than ourselves. True professional maturity demands that we do as much. This book is the first of a new breed, in both its comprehensiveness and explicitness. The authors are to be congratulated not only for their ideas but for demonstrating that we are indeed growing up.

Audrey L. Holland, Ph.D.
University of Pittsburgh

PREFACE

Together, we have practiced speech-language pathology for 26 years. During that time, personally we have seen many aphasic patients for language treatment and we have also trained many students to work with these individuals. Along the way we have been struck by the relative lack of research-based information about aphasia treatment.

Until recently, there have been few research studies supporting the efficacy of language treatment. Although speech-language pathologists believed that aphasic patients benefited from treatment and patients testified to that effect, there was little hard research evidence to support the claim. Several efficacy studies have been done in the last decade, with the conclusion that treatment is efficacious. The problem is what kind of treatment, for the studies did not describe it in sufficient detail that clinicians in the field could replicate it.

Several methods that have been described in the literature have provided little research data supporting the idea that they accrue benefits above and beyond those expected through natural recovery processes. Clinicians need to know that the methods they use with patients are efficacious.

Although materials abound for use with aphasic patients, their purposes are frequently not clearly specified and their level of difficulty is not defined. Clinicians in the field would benefit from materials that are designed for specific purposes, whose content is systematically organized, and whose difficulty levels are gradually increased. They could then see the rationale behind how and why materials are developed and how to plan additional ones.

To meet these needs in an approach to aphasia rehabilitation is the goal of this book. We wanted to provide a comprehensive treatment approach that would present efficacy data and would offer materials that had been designed for and used with the aphasic subjects treated.

The guidelines for Language-Oriented Treatment (LOT) provided are sufficiently specific that they can be reliably followed by clinicians and replicated. However, they are flexible enough to support individualized treatment programs in which the patient's behavior and progress form the basis for treatment focus and direction. The guidelines are just that—guidelines, not prescriptions. They allow clinicians to make informed decisions about each aphasic patient's individualized treatment plan.

To undertake such a large endeavor required the efforts of many people whose contributions we gratefully acknowledge. This work was supported in part by grant DM 324 Language Therapy and Recovery from Aphasia from the Ontario Ministry of Health and by a grant from The University of Western Ontario Foundation, Inc. We would like to thank both the clinicians who provided treatment and the patients and their families for participating in the treatment study. In addition, the impeccable computer work of Doug Link from the Social Sciences Computing Laboratory and the statistical advice of Allan Donner were invaluable. Jane Bartram provided helpful comments on early drafts of the manuscript. For a well-prepared manuscript, we extend our gratitude to Shirley Smith and Linda Platt.

Cynthia M. Shewan, Ph.D.
Donna L. Bandur, M.Cl.Sc.
London, Ontario

Chapter 1

Introducing Language-Oriented Treatment

The management of aphasic patients is a complex undertaking that involves the coordinated efforts of a rehabilitation team representing several disciplines. As members of one of these disciplines, speech-language pathologists share with other health care professionals the goal of rehabilitating aphasic patients to their best possible level of functioning. To accomplish that goal the best quality speech-language services available must be provided. This means that speech-language pathologists must use language treatment programs that have proved to be efficacious and that have been described in sufficient detail so that they can be reliably utilized by practicing clinicians rather than restricted to the designers' use alone. To foster use of such programs and to make them time-efficient for clinicians, examples of appropriate treatment materials and suggestions for constructing others are needed. It was these needs for adequately described and demonstrated efficacious treatment methods with accompanying treatment materials that prompted the development of Language-Oriented Treatment (LOT) (Shewan, 1977).

THE HISTORY OF APHASIA TREATMENT

Although it is clearly beyond the scope of this book to review completely the history of aphasia treatment, a short review will provide a perspective from which to view the current state. (The reader interested in pursuing this topic is referred to Shewan, 1985, LaPointe, 1983, and Riese, 1947, for more detailed accounts.)

Little in the way of orthodox treatments appeared until the beginning of the twentieth century. Prior to this herbs and potions were used as well as remedies affecting the vascular system, such as leeching, blistering, and cautery. A few case reports including language information appeared in the early 1900s (Mills, 1904; Franz, 1906, 1924), and several studies focused on aphasia as a result of trauma following World War I (Frazier and Ingham, 1920; Weisenburg and McBride, 1935). The early history of aphasia emphasized treatment very little, although these studies, which did address the area, raised questions about the nature and efficacy of language treatment that remained unanswered for many years. Researchers at this stage reported that treatment was effective, although they did not prove it.

The post World War II years witnessed a surge of interest in aphasia rehabilitation that was focused on reintegrating the young veterans into life's mainstream. Rehabilitation programs spread throughout the United States and included speech services as part of the overall program. Many programs included academic subjects, reading, writing, arithmetic, and spelling and drew content and personnel from the education field, since re-education was the underlying theme of rehabilitation.

Because of the effects on and changes in personality following traumatic brain injury, psychotherapy groups became a part of rehabilitation programs (Backus, 1952; Blackman, 1950). Usually designed as support groups, they reportedly positively influenced both communication and personality adjustment of patients (Aronson, Shatin, and Cook, 1956; Blackman and Tureen, 1948). Improved communication fostered better personality adjustment that, in turn, promoted better communication.

During this time the question of the efficacy of treatment was raised many times; however, most of the supportive evidence was anecdotal and lacking in statistical confirmation. Wepman's (1951) and Eisenson's (1949) work added important information about the positive effects of treatment but dealt almost exclusively with traumatic aphasia.

A shift in the aphasic patient population from trauma to cerebrovascular accident (CVA) occurred in the 1950s, with the result that the effects of rehabilitation, including speech and language, were extended to this group (Godfrey and Douglass, 1959; Marks, Taylor, and Rusk, 1957). Schuell's work of the 1950s and 1960s (Schuell, Jenkins, and Jiménez-Pabón, 1964) extended knowledge about the assessment and treatment of aphasia; one of its strong and enduring influences was stimulation treatment. A landmark study was Vignolo's (1964) report of the positive effects of language treatment when it was initiated early and lasted at least 6 months. However, this work was counterbalanced by Sarno, Silverman, and Sands's (1970) report of no significant treatment benefits for a group of severely impaired aphasic patients. The latter finding, overgeneralized to the entire aphasic population, was frequently used as evidence that speech treatment was not efficacious.

Therefore, the 1970s started with the case for language treatment in hot debate. Darley (1972), in his classic article, challenged the profession to answer three important questions: (1) Does language treatment provide significant positive benefits beyond those expected due to spontaneous recovery? (2) Are the treatment gains worth the time, effort, and cost incurred in achieving them? and (3) Which methods of language treatment are most effective?

The next decade concentrated on research that would attempt to lay the efficacy question to rest. By 1975, Holland reported that little progress had been made. She also suggested that answers to the question of efficacy, defined as "the power to effect," could be approached through single case studies and small sample research studies designed to determine whether speech-language pathologists were helping patients and what they were doing that helped.

MODERN EFFICACY STUDIES

The question of the efficacy of language treatment is a difficult one to study. There are methodological complications combined with an enormous time commitment. The optimal experimental design calls for a randomized no-treatment control group, which serves as a control for natural recovery. This design then requires withholding treatment, which presents ethical problems (Shewan and Kertesz, 1984). This issue aside, there is also that of whether the control group really remains "untreated," as the patients themselves, relatives, friends, and perhaps nurses attempt to assist language recovery (Gloning, Trappl, Heiss, and Quatember, 1976; Griffith, 1970; Riese, 1947; Weisenburg and McBride, 1935). For a more complete review of the efficacy issue and related studies, the reader is referred to Shewan (1985) and Darley (1982).

Using nonrandomized control groups is one avenue that has been adopted by several researchers studying efficacy (Basso, Capitani, and Vignolo, 1979; Basso, Faglioni, and Vignolo, 1975; Deal and Deal, 1978; Hagen, 1973; Shewan and Kertesz, 1984). Either control groups can be matched with the experimental group at the outset, or statistical means, such as analysis of covariance, can be used to account for any group imbalances. Results from the aforementioned studies designed in this way have uniformly yielded positive results, favoring greater language recovery in treated patients.

Several additional studies, without using control groups, have also provided evidence toward solving the efficacy issue. If a 3-month period post stroke is used as representing the time during which spontaneous recovery occurs (Sarno and Levita, 1971) and treatment effects are examined either excluding this period or using subjects who initiated treatment after this period, the data support the positive effects for language treatment (Broida, 1977; Butfield and Zangwill, 1946; Dabul and Hanson, 1975; Prins, Snow, and Wagenaar, 1978; Sands, Sarno, and Shankweiler, 1969; Sefer, 1973; Smith, Champoux, Leri, London, and Muraski, 1972; Wertz et al., 1978; Wertz et al., 1981). It can be argued that the perfect experimental study remains to be done and that the studies cited vary in the degree to which they have met the standards of a rigorous clinical trials study. However, their consistency in reporting positive treatment effects for those patients who received treatment supports Darley's conclusion (1982) " . . . the foregoing collage of studies . . . collectively provides a series of answers and together lays our doubt about efficacy to rest" (p.175).

TYPES OF APHASIA TREATMENT

As seen from the literature review given, aphasia treatment has been provided to aphasic patients for several decades. Despite this history and almost two dozen efficacy studies, the type of treatment provided has rarely been described or uniformly carried out. The truth of Prins and coworkers' (1978) statement, ". . . the exact content of the therapy sessions was highly variable, dependent on the patient, the treatment centre, and the speech therapist involved" (p. 19), makes it difficult, therefore, for a clinician to employ these efficacious treatment programs.

Group treatment, popular in the 1940s and 1950s, gave way to a focus on individual treatment. The relative effectiveness of these two delivery methods was examined recently by Wertz and colleagues (1981). Both individually treated and group-treated subject groups made significant language gains, with few differences apparent between the groups. Where differences did exist, they favored individual treatment. Programmed instruction was used in several studies, but a comparison of this approach with traditional treatment is limited to the Sarno and associates study (1970), which used only global aphasic patients. That no differences between treatment types were found may say more about the severity of the language impairment than the type of treatment.

Some treatment programs described in the literature in the last few years include Response-Contingent Small-Step Performance-Based Communication Intervention (Bollinger and Stout, 1976), Base-10 Programmed Stimulation (LaPointe, 1977), A Procedure Manual in Speech Pathology with Brain-damaged Adults (Keenan, 1975), and PACE Therapy (Davis and Wilcox, 1981). The unfortunate shortcoming of these methods is that efficacy data are lacking. Some additional specialized methods of treatment have been described in a sufficiently detailed manner to be replicable across clinicians (Melodic Intonation Therapy by Sparks, 1981, and Sparks, Helm, and Albert, 1974; Visual Action Therapy by Helm and Benson, 1978, and Helm-Estabrooks, Fitzpatrick, and Barresi, 1982; Visual Communication (VIC) by Gardner, Zurif, Berry, and Baker, 1976; and Voluntary Control of Involuntary Utterances by Helm and Barresi, 1980). However, these methods are applicable to only specific groups of aphasic patients.

APPROACHES TO LANGUAGE TREATMENT

Language treatment for the aphasic patient has taken many different forms. Some methods, such as Schuell and associates' (1964) stimulation treatment, were designed to be adaptable to aphasic patients in general. Other methods, such as Melodic Intonation Therapy (Sparks, 1981), apply only to patients who meet specific language profile criteria.

Treatments vary in their underlying philosophies. Some derive directly from the aphasiologist's belief of what aphasia represents. For those who believed that aphasia was a loss of language, rehabilitation approaches focused on relearning or re-education. This was common among treatment programs after World War II (Corbin, 1951; Peacher, 1946; Wepman, 1951). Among current treatments, Base-10 Programmed Stimulation (LaPointe, 1977) emphasizes a relearning approach. When responses are established at a criterion level (accurate, complete, prompt responses with scores of 15 on the Porch Index of Communicative Ability [PICA] multidimensional scoring system), the stimuli are changed and the patient practices with these until the criterion is again reached. The aphasic patient is learning responses to presented stimuli. The re-education approach is also incorporated into treatments based on the linguistic regression hypothesis that language breaks down in the reverse order to its acquisition.

However, that aphasia does not represent a loss of language has been well documented in the literature. For example, Schuell and co-workers (1964) and Jenkins, Jiménez-Pabón, Shaw, and Sefer (1975) have frequently referred to the reduction in the availability of vocabulary to the aphasic patient, but they are not of the impression that specific vocabulary is lost to the patient. Howes and Geschwind (1964) reported data indicating that the aphasic individual has a potentially limitless vocabulary although he or she does demonstrate a tendency to use frequently occurring lexical items rather than rare ones. If the language impairment in aphasia does not represent a loss, then treatment cannot be viewed primarily as a re-education program. This view is supported by Schuell and co-workers (1964) and Pöeck (1982) who stated that aphasia language treatment is neither retraining language, teaching language to an adult as a second language, nor teaching language to a child who has not yet acquired it. It is assumed that the clinician is not teaching new material to the aphasic patient but rather is attempting to improve, reorganize, or maximize the efficiency of the impaired language system.

Another school of thought regarding language treatment views aphasia as representing a reduced efficiency of functioning. Perhaps two subgroups of thought should be distinguished in this approach: (1) The language system is impaired and therefore operates less efficiently and perhaps differently from normal and (2) access to the language system is cut off, thereby resulting in disturbed language performance. Treatment approaches aligned with this view of aphasia generally attempt to stimulate language processing in the patient. However, their neuropsychological or neurophysiological effects are yet undetermined because methods do not exist for differentiating whether

1. Treatment stimulates the repair of old processes-pathways and functions as remediation.
2. Treatment teaches the patient new ways to approach a problem or new strategies to attack the problem and functions as compensation.
3. Treatment functions to reorganize brain function by developing new programs-pathways.
4. Treatment establishes old functions in new brain areas.
5. Treatment serves to facilitate right hemisphere functioning.

Other differences in therapies relate to the content included. Wepman (1953) first expressed little concern for the content of treatment, advocating stimulation and facilitation of language in general, whereas his later work (1972) emphasized the stimulation of ideas rather than language. He emphasized a good client-clinician relationship and a good communication environment as being important to patient improvement. Other approaches have given more attention to what is presented in treatment, indicating that the content is important. Response-Contingent Small-Step Performance-Based Communicative Intervention (Bollinger and Stout, 1976) uses hierarchical steps that increase the level of item difficulty within and across tasks. For example, high frequency items would be presented in a naming task prior to low frequency items.

Information about psycholinguistics, the processing and use of language by normal subjects, has been utilized in some aspects of training for the last 20 years. Scargill (1954) emphasized the importance of psycholinguistic concepts in teaching aphasic patients, for example, teaching language patterns rather than teaching the lexicon alone. Despite an interest in psycholinguistics by aphasia researchers and clinicians, LOT is the first comprehensive description of a treatment approach using psycholinguistic information.

LANGUAGE-ORIENTED TREATMENT (LOT)

Philosophy and Rationale

Language-Oriented Treatment has it roots in a particular view about aphasia that maintains that the language system itself is impaired or disturbed as well as that access to it potentially is disturbed. Therefore, aphasia does not represent simply a loss of language or impaired access to an otherwise normal language system; rather, aspects of the system, phonological, semantic, syntactic, or any combination of these, are impaired. Evidence to support this view comes from many sources, some of the most potent being Zurif and his colleagues' work (Zurif and Caramazza, 1976; Zurif, Caramazza and Myerson, 1972; Zurif, Green, Caramazza and Goodenough, 1976; Whitehouse, Caramazza, and Zurif, 1978) with agrammatic aphasic patients. These patients were impaired not only in their ability to produce or construct grammatical sentences but also in their underlying knowledge about basic grammatical relationships. Zurif and co-workers (1972, 1976) found that patients with Broca's aphasia paid little attention to function words when analyzing the meaning of a sentence and did not group members of linguistic constituents in ways characteristic of normal subjects. For example, given a sentence such as "My brother hit a home run," normal subjects indicated close relations between nouns and their modifiers, for example, "brother" and "my" and "home run" and "a," but the aphasic subjects did not. This suggested an impairment in the syntactic system itself.

Data have also demonstrated that aphasic patients' semantic knowledge appears to be disrupted. The scope of their semantic categories did not coincide with normal subjects' semantic category boundaries (L'hermittee, Dérouensné, and Lecours, 1971) and they did not make the same distinctions among semantic features as did normal adults (Zurif and Caramazza, 1976; Zurif, Caramazza, Myerson, and Galvin, 1974).

That there is impaired access to aspects of the language system is demonstrated by the Broca's aphasic patient who can write a word but not say it or by the patient who can spell a word orally but not write it (Kinsbourne and Rosenfield, 1974; Rothi and Heilman, 1981).

The frequently reduced scores and the increased latency of various types of responses in aphasic patients demonstrate their reduced efficiency in processing language. Since aphasia does involve reduced efficiency, one of the goals of LOT is to increase the patient's efficiency of processing language both receptively and expressively. However, reduced efficiency of operation does not appear to explain all aspects of aphasic language impairment.

In addition to impairment of the language system, aphasia also involves a disturbance to processing mechanisms for understanding and producing language. For example, an aphasic patient may fail to understand a passive sentence because of processing it like an active one, perhaps as a result of confusion between the agent and object in the sentence (Shewan and Canter, 1971). One of the ways that processing problems may be circumvented is via teaching aphasic patients to employ a different strategy to approach a problem or to use a cueing system to aid processing (Shewan, 1976b; Whitney, 1975). For example, having the aphasic patient delay before responding has been found as one effective strategy for aiding word retrieval difficulties (Marshall, 1976). That training does not merely teach trained material but generalizes to processes involved in processing language has been suggested by Wiegel-Crump and Koenigsknecht (1973). They showed that aphasic patients made gains in naming ability for both trained and untrained semantic categories. Training appeared not merely to be teaching forgotten vocabulary items but to be positively influencing the aphasics' word retrieval processes. These principles are incorporated into LOT.

LOT views the language content of treatment as important. Treatment is more than providing indiscriminant stimulation. Because language is not lost, the goal is not strictly retraining or re-education. However, the language system is impaired and the content of treatment is directed toward those impaired modalities and at levels that are appropriate to the degree of impairment. Whurr's findings (1983) that aphasic patients made significantly greater gains with treatment focused on their deficit areas compared with patients whose treatment emphasized their retained areas of function support the importance of the content of treatment. LOT's goals are to facilitate improved efficiency, reorganization, and/or the establishment of functions in homologous brain areas so that language processing operates at its best possible level.

In order to plan content appropriately, treatment materials and their progression in difficulty should reflect current knowledge about how patients process language. To that end, LOT is based on information and data gathered from the fields of speech-language pathology, linguistics, psycholinguistics, and neuropsychology. Because content of this approach reflects knowledge about language, its organization, its processing, and its recovery from brain damage, it was classified as a psycholinguistic one and thus was termed Language-Oriented Treatment.

How treatment is approached methodologically is another important treatment issue. This is to be distinguished from the content of treatment. Approaches based on learning principles, usually operant procedures, fell into disrepute in the 1970s as there seemed to be some confusion between treatment content and methodology. Programmed treatment was viewed as synonymous with operant conditioning, with a nonpatient focus, and often with a rote learning orientation. However, programming is not the process itself of treatment. As Holland (1975) so well states ". . . programming is what makes the process accessible and replicable enough for systematic study lending to possible answers to that why . . ." (p. 151). Therefore, the methodology of treatment can be based on learning principles without sacrificing the importance of both content and individualized treatment programs.

Because every aphasic patient comes to treatment with a different pattern of language impairment and a different environmental background, training should account for his or her interests and level of functioning. The topics discussed in treatment would vary among patients—a farmer and a business executive are likely to have different interest levels with regard to the varieties of cattle feed on the market. Difficulty level of material would also vary—one patient may be able to communicate with single words only, whereas another may be functioning at a sentence level in production. Eisenson (1971) capsulizes the idea well: "The best techniques are those which are designed for the individual patient" (p. 1266).

Content

As indicated in the previous section, the language content of LOT is considered very important; that is to say, what language materials and tasks the clinician presents are important to a patient's progress. Training in the deficit language areas and training with language content at an appropriate difficulty level are important. The general goal of treatment is to improve the patient's communication to its premorbid level or as close to that level as possible. For severely impaired patients, an alternate system or augmentative system to oral language may be required.

To specify the content of LOT more specifically, the communication system was divided into five modalities. These served as the major content divisions of LOT: (1) auditory processing, (2) visual processing, (3) gestural and combined gestural-verbal communication, (4) oral expression, and (5) graphic expression (Fig. 1–1). The modalities are considered to

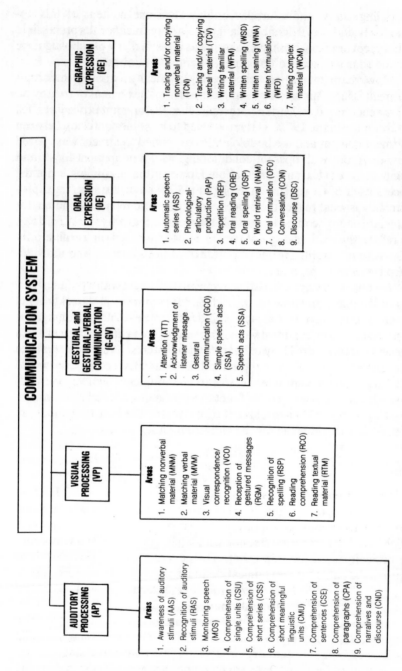

Figure 1–1. A schematic model of the language modalities and areas within these modalities that comprise the communication system.

be mutually exclusive and nonoverlapping to facilitate planning therapy and recording data. Training in any modality is designed to involve that modality (1) exclusively when possible and practicable or (2) primarily with another modality involved in a minor capacity and at a sufficiently easy level that it does not interfere with performance. For example, identification of objects named by the examiner is classified as an auditory comprehension task and is therefore included in the auditory processing modality. It is recognized that the visual modality is involved in perception of the objects and that some form of pointing (motor) response is required. However, the communication aspect of the task is one of auditory processing. The guiding principle here is that the activity should emphasize that modality being trained and make minimal demands from any other modality.

Each of the five modalities is divided into areas, one or more of which may be appropriate to include in training (Fig. 1–1). The areas specify in greater detail content aspects within the modality. Again, to assist in coding and replication of treatment, the areas are mutually exclusive and collectively encompass the entire modality. By way of example, the auditory processing modality is divided into nine areas: (1) awareness of auditory stimuli, (2) recognition of auditory stimuli, (3) monitoring speech, (4) comprehension of single units, (5) comprehension of short series, (6) comprehension of short meaningful linguistic units, (7) comprehension of sentences, (8) comprehension of paragraphs, and (9) comprehension of narratives and discourse. In the chapters describing treatment for each modality, detailed material for each area has been included outlining the task-difficulty hierarchies, stimulus corpus that might be involved in training tasks, specific variables to consider controlling because of their known influence on aphasic patients' processing, and the response corpus in the case of the expressive modalities. Where the literature provided information regarding difficulty of items within an area, the stimuli or responses have been organized into hierarchies, with the easiest material listed first. To highlight these hierarchies they have been enclosed in □ (boxes) throughout the text. When research was unavailable to indicate a ranking according to difficulty level, either a hierarchy was suggested only or the stimuli were not rank ordered. These listings were not enclosed in boxes to differentiate them from the previous ones.

A description of the general activities included within each area is provided. This gives the clinician a frame of reference for the intent of the training, the types of activities that would be included, and the goal of these activities. Following the description is an example of a specific activity that would fall within the area. Treatment materials and activities for several difficulty levels for each area for each modality are provided in the chapter following the description of each modality. The difficulty levels included in each area having been coded as beginning, intermediate, or advanced. This should further assist the clinician in selecting an appropriate level of task difficulty for the patient. Suggestions for creating additional materials are also provided. These materials are meant to suggest possibilities for training to the clinician but are not considered to be exhaustive.

The purpose of specifying the language content of LOT is to enable the clinician to administer treatment addressed to an aphasic patient's specific speech and language deficits, to select materials at a level appropriate to these respective deficits in various language modalities, and to present material in steps that increase in difficulty using language materials arranged hierarchically according to difficulty, the difficulty being based, when possible, on psycholinguistic information about aphasics' processing of language.

Because every patient is different and has different interests, LOT programs are individualized. Using a systematic methodology does not preclude individualized content in training. To select content for training the clinician should include information from standardized test performance, clinical observation of the patient, and a case history. Information from these three sources is used to select the modalities requiring treatment. Because communication primarily involves speaking and listening in our everyday world, these modalities are most often selected for training, as they are potentially the most beneficial and closest to the mode of premorbid functioning. As well, they are always impaired in aphasia, although to differing degrees across aphasic types. The remaining three modalities may or may not be selected for training. Generally, visual processing will be included at some point during the training program and the extent of graphic expression will depend on the overall degree of impairment as well as the patient's premorbid proficiency, frequency of use, and interest in pursuing it.

When the modalities requiring treatment have been selected, the clinician then selects goals within each modality. Generally three or four major goals would be selected. For example, three major goals for a particular patient might be (1) to improve auditory comprehension of sentences, (2) to improve word-finding abilities, and (3) to improve oral formulation of phrases and simple sentences. It is unwise to select only one goal, since treatment sessions are usually one hour in length and working on the same aspect of treatment for an entire hour might be fatiguing. Goals having been selected, the clinician then chooses the relevant specific areas in which training will take place. For example, when working on the goal to improve auditory comprehension of sentences, the clinician would select the areas of comprehension of short linguistic units, comprehension of sentences, or both as the area or areas for training.

The specific activities in training are left to the clinician's judgment. Usually there will be several options based on the interests of the patient, the level of functioning, and the nature of the goal to be accomplished. For example, activities appropriate for improving auditory comprehension of sentences include (1) selecting an appropriate picture to match a sentence read to the patient, (2) working on a sentence completion activity, or (3) following directions, answering yes-no questions, or both.

Both the clinician and the patient may desire to use several activities within one treatment session or across treatment sessions to achieve a specific goal. This will enhance the interest of the patient in activities and will also build some stimulus generalization into the program.

The clinician should design training activities that are at an appropriate level of difficulty for the patient. Because this aspect of LOT will be described more fully in a subsequent section, it is mentioned only briefly to provide continuity in describing the content of treatment. The level at which the patient makes errors at a rate of 20 to 30 percent on a formalized test or with in-depth clinical testing would be an appropriate starting level of difficulty. For example, if a patient's error rate for understanding sentences was 20 to 30 percent, it would be appropriate to start at this level of training for auditory comprehension.

The next content question facing the clinician is what types of stimuli would be appropriate to use for training. The hierarchies of difficulty, based on the performance of groups of aphasic patients, assist in these decisions. Since these hierarchies are reflective of group performance, the same hierarchy may not hold for all aphasic patients. By gathering baseline data, the clinician can determine each individual's particular hierarchy of difficulty and can select content using this knowledge. Following up on the previous example, the clinician would select several types of sentence forms for the auditory comprehension portion of treatment.

Methodology of Training

In addition to considerations of content of training (the "what" of treatment), the clinician is also concerned with the methodology or administration of that training (the "how" of treatment).

The methodological approach selected for LOT arises from learning theory, operant paradigms in particular. However, the goal is *not* operant conditioning; that is, the learning of a specific response upon presentation of an antecedent event (stimulus) followed by reinforcing consequences. In LOT stimuli are presented, the client makes a response, and the clinician provides feedback. However, the learning of specific stimulus-response bonds is not the goal. In LOT the same stimuli are not used over and over again until the client learns them to a criterion of 80 to 90 percent correct; rather, different stimuli at a comparable level of processing difficulty are presented to elicit responses. Knowledge of results is provided so the clinician and client know how well the client is able to process at this level and, consequently, when to proceed to the next level of difficulty. The verbal reinforcement by the clinician to the client is not thought to be the prime determiner of success. Rather the method provides opportunities for patients to access and to process language material at a level appropriate to their abilities. This processing provides practice and reorganizational opportunities so that the neurphysiological mechanism can improve or appropriately alter its functioning. This may happen by increasing efficiency, developing alternate pathways or networks, or repairing impaired pathways. The stimuli presented may be auditory, visual (verbal or nonverbal), tactile, gestural, or combinations of the above. The response that the client makes might be gestural, oral, or graphic. The clinician provides feedback as to the correctness of the client's response and may provide qualitative evaluation of the response. For example, the clinician might say, "You got the correct answers with only one repetition this time; you needed two last time."

This type of methodological paradigm was selected because of its perceived advantages administratively, professionally, and scientifically. It specifies a systematic administrative approach that can be replicated by clinicians in an individual center or practice and across centers or institutions. In a given center this allows the administration to gather important information for quality assurance and about their service provision. Among centers and in the profession it allows the opportunity for the widespread provision of efficacious services to aphasic clients. Scientifically, it allows researchers and clinicians to gather data on a widespread basis to provide information that will help to answer questions about aphasia treatment and that will provide impetus for designing studies to investigate further questions.

Difficulty Level

LOT specifies that associated with each area selected for training is an appropriate starting difficulty level. This is the level at which the patient's error rate is approximately 20 to 30 percent. It can be determined from standardized test performance, from criterion-referenced tests designed by the clinician, from gathering baseline data, or from combinations of these.

Baseline Data. Because standardized test performance data may be insufficient to establish a starting difficulty level, gathering baseline data will be discussed. Baseline information will also be used to establish the difficulty hierarchies through which the client will progress. A separate hierarchy is necessary for each area within each modality selected for training. To provide continuity, the previous example of comprehending sentences will be used. The clinician needs to know which sentence forms to include in treatment and what their relative degrees of difficulty are for a particular patient. Chapter 2 provides a difficulty hierarchy from which to start. A test can be constructed to contain five examples of each of six sentence types. Results from administration of this criterion-referenced test can be used to construct the difficulty hierarchy. Those sentence forms on which the patient's error rate is 20 to 30 percent can be used to start treatment. The other sentence types are rank ordered in ascending difficulty of training as criterion is reached on previous types. If, from these baseline data, the clinician determines that the aphasic patient is following an already established hierarchy (e.g., the sentence type comprehension hierarchy in Chapter 2), then baseline testing will not need to be repeated as additional sentence forms are selected for training. If this is not the case, however, additional baseline testing will be necessary.

Baseline data are also needed when establishing or using a cueing system with a patient. A cueing system may help a patient to process levels of language that he or she would be otherwise unable to manage. A frequent occurrence is the use of cueing to assist with word retrieval difficulties. Research has established that there are several cues that can help to elicit a response (see Chapter 8). Baseline data are necessary to determine which cues are most effective for a particular patient. As facility in word retrieval is regained, cues that were initially effective may cease to become so or cues that were not effective may now be appropriate to use. Therefore, periodic baselines or probes will be necessary to insure consistent use of effective cues.

In cases in which there are several response possibilities, the clinician may need to gather baseline data to determine the progression of responses. Criterion for a correct response may be repetition at one level and spontaneous production at another level. Of course, the clinician may know a priori what the hierarchy is, thus eliminating the need for a baseline. Clinical judgment determines whether a baseline is necessary.

A general rule for gathering baseline data may be helpful. If you are starting treatment and do not have data available to organize a difficulty hierarchy or if you are training an area and need information about the hierarchy of difficulty of the stimuli or cues you are presenting, or the responses you are expecting, collect baseline data to establish the hierarchy of difficulty for the patient. This will also have the effect of organizing the levels along which to proceed in training.

Increasing the Difficulty Level. Activities in LOT are presented in blocks of 10 stimulus items each (Fig. 1–2). The patient much achieve correct responses for the ten items of at least 70 percent to achieve criterion. He or she should achieve this 70 percent criterion on two consecutive

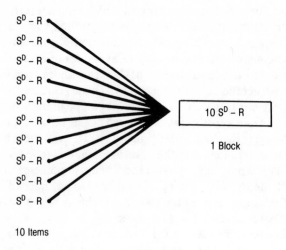

Figure 1-2.   Ten stimulus items (S^D) and their responses (R) constitute one block.

blocks before advancing to the next difficulty level. Task difficulty is increased gradually using this method, as shown in Figure 1–3. If the patient does not achieve 70 percent correct, the same stimulus block (10 stimulus items) is repeated. If, with repetition, the patient still does not achieve 70 percent, the difficulty level of the task is reduced, as shown in Figure 1–4. If the patient cannot perform with a repetition of the reduced difficulty task, then the task should be terminated. It becomes obvious that the activity is beyond the level at which the patient can function (Fig. 1–4).

Figure 1–5 combines previous ones to show the clinician how to arrange the blocks of stimuli for any given activity. When criterion is reached on two blocks of stimuli, the difficulty of the material increases. When criterion is not reached, a repetition of the task is given. If the patient is still unable to perform, the difficulty level of the task is reduced.

A 70 percent criterion level was chosen rather than the 80 percent level more frequently used in speech-language pathology. One reason for this choice was the small number of stimuli (10) in each block. If larger blocks were used, an 80 percent criterion level might have been appropriate. A 70 percent criterion allowed the patient to make two or three errors per block before considering the need to repeat the task. To obtain that one additional correct response, which corresponds to a 10 percent increase, may have taken more time than would have been profitable to spend in treatment. The 70 percent criterion appeared to allow a greater amount of flexibility in the LOT program.

Sometimes the nature of the treatment does not neatly fit into providing blocks of 10 stimulus items or trials. For example, if conversation is the

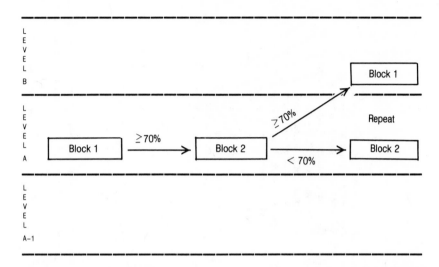

Figure 1–3. This figure shows the progression of treatment, starting at an arbitrary level of difficulty termed Level A. If the patient achieves the 70 percent criterion on Block 1, Block 2 stimuli are presented. If criterion is reached, the patient advances to the next level of difficulty, Level B. If criterion is not reached, Block 2 is repeated. Level A–1 represents a reduced level of difficulty from Level A.

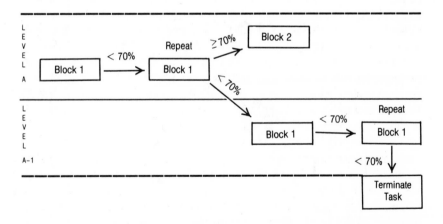

Figure 1–4. This figure shows the sequence of events when the 70 percent criterion is not reached. Starting at an arbitrary level of difficulty, Level A, the patient does not achieve criterion on Block 1; therefore, it is repeated. If the patient does not achieve criterion with the repetition, the level of difficulty is reduced to Level A–1. A block of stimuli are presented and failure to achieve criterion results in a repetition, which in turn results in termination of the task if once again criterion is not reached.

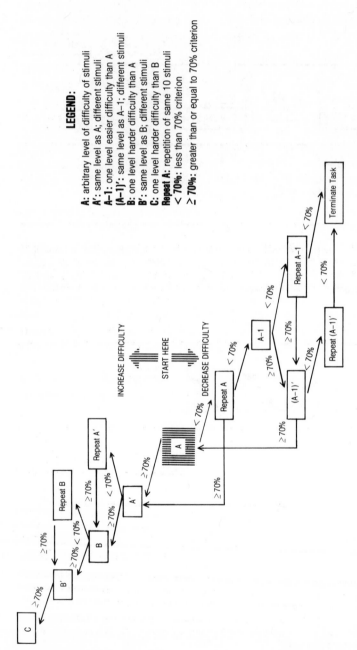

LEGEND:

A: arbitrary level of difficulty of stimuli
A′: same level as A; different stimuli
A−1: one level easier difficulty than A
(A−1)′: same level as A−1; different stimuli
B: one level harder difficulty than A
B′: same level as B; different stimuli
C: one level harder difficulty than B
Repeat A: repetition of same 10 stimuli
< 70%: less than 70% criterion
≥ 70%: greater than or equal to 70% criterion

Figure 1–5. Summary model of the administration of LOT. The starting point is A. A block of 10 items is presented to the aphasic patient. If 70 percent or more correct responses is achieved, the clinician proceeds to A′, another block of 10 items at the same difficulty level as A. If 70 percent or more is achieved, the level of difficulty is increased and the clinician proceeds to B to initiate another cycle. If less than 70 percent correct responses is achieved at A, the clinician repeats A. If 70 percent or more is achieved, the clinician proceeds to A′; if not, the level of difficulty is reduced and the clinician regresses to A−1. If the level of difficulty is reduced one level and repeated with less than 70 percent success, the task is terminated.

response it may not be appropriate to spend 10 training sessions at this level. Therefore, the clinician may specify 10 five-minute conversational segments as representing a block. In this way, if the 70 percent criterion is not met it will be determined in 1 or 2 training sessions rather than 10. The modality of graphic expression may require this type of modification at times.

Using 70 percent as a criterion level is suggested for LOT. However, the performance of an individual patient may indicate that a higher criterion level would be more appropriate. If a patient always needs repetition of both blocks at a given level of difficulty and drops considerably below 70 percent at the next difficulty level, it may be appropriate to use an 80 percent criterion level. Although the data presented in this volume used the 70 percent criterion level in the majority of cases, occasional exceptions were made when warranted. The clinician should feel free to make them with his or her patients when appropriate.

Increasing difficulty necessitates the elaboration of three terms: cueing, criterion response, and branching.

Cueing. A patient may not be able to produce a response completely independently. Therefore, a series of cues or prompts may assist in eliciting the target response. Some familiar cues are repeating the stimulus, providing the first sound of the word, and so on. As the patient becomes more proficient, this support from the clinician can be reduced and may be transferred so that the patient can provide his or her own cues (self-cueing). Altering cue support is one way of increasing the level of difficulty in LOT.

The general goal is to teach aphasic patients strategies or cues that they can eventually use as aids in language processing. Since aphasia training is not designed to teach responses but to improve efficiency or to improve an impaired mechanism, providing strategies for the patient can aid performance and increase independence from the clinician. For example, with word retrieval problems, the idea is not to eradicate them since they will continue unless language recovers completely. Rather the goal is to teach the patient how to deal with the problem when it occurs. One way is to provide strategies that can be used to elicit the word, such as thinking of the first sound of the word, gesturing the action, and so forth. The aphasic patient may already use strategies but may be unaware of them or unaware that they are effective. In this case the clinician's goal is for the patient to recognize personal strategies and to encourage their consistent use. On other occasions the clinician may have to devise strategies for the patient, provide practice using them, and later transfer their initiation to the patient.

This progression involves four major phases:

1. Determining which cues or strategies are effective for the patient.

2. Increasing the patient's awareness of the effective cues.
3. Transferring initiation of the cues or strategies from the clinician to the patient.
4. Increasing the patient's use of effective strategies or cues.

The material below incorporates the suggestions of Berman and Peale (1967). A detailed outline of a cue hierarchy, emphasizing the four phases, is presented to familiarize the clinician with how it might apply in LOT. The examples are of word-retrieval or naming activities because they represent a universal problem in aphasia and a frequently trained area in treatment.

Cue Hierarchy

1. Establish the effectiveness of different cues. Collect *baseline* data.
   Sources of information:
   • Test information
   • Client's use of cues
   • Spouse information
   • Criterion-referenced test
2. The clinician provides cues. This stage is designed to increase the patient's *awareness* of cues. The patient is informed of the purpose of cueing and of which cues are most effective for him or her. The clinician initiates cueing, selects the cues, and provides the cues. At first the clinician provides the most potent or effective cue and/or as many others as are necessary to elicit a target response.
   (i) Most effective cue; for example, "It starts with /s/."
   (ii) Additional cues.
3. The clinician gives instruction to use a specific cue. It is not the most effective one. Additional cues are provided as necessary to elicit a target response.
   (i) Use a cue; for example, "I will tell you a related word. It is _____."
   (ii) Provides additional cues.
4. The clinician writes all cues down and the patient selects the one for the clinician to provide. This is the first stage of *transferring* cueing from the clinician to the patient. The patient initiates the cueing and the clinician provides the cues. In (i) the clinician selects the cues; in (ii) the patient selects them.
   (i) The patient is given the three most effective cues and selects from these. The clinician provides the selected cue.
   (ii) The patient selects which cues are appropriate from a wider array, and then indicates which cue the clinician should provide.
5. The clinician asks the patient to self-cue. This is a second stage of *transfer*. The cues are available in written form if necessary. The clinician prompts the patient for each item. The patient now initiates, selects, and provides the cues.
   (i) The clinician may prompt the patient by asking "What can you do to help?" or "What helps you?"
   (ii) As the patient is able to use self-cues, the clinician provides fewer prompts.
6. The patient is responsible for the cueing process (initiating cueing, selecting cues, self-cueing). The clinician provides instruction about cue-

ing only at the beginning of the treatment activity. This is the first stage of *effective use* of cues.

- (i) The clinician provides instruction initially in the activity, "When you have trouble, think about what helps you."
- (ii) The patient initiates at least one cue. The clinician adds others if necessary.

7. The patient initiates cueing without instruction. This is the second stage of *effective use* of cues.

- (i) The patient uses more than one cue as necessary to elicit a target response. If cueing does not elicit the response, the clinician provides additional cues and/or the response. The goal is to have the patient use cues effectively.

8. The patient initiates cueing and provides his or her own cues independently. This is the last stage of *effective cueing*. Many patients find it helpful to have their cues available as key words on a 3 × 5 card which they carry in a pocket or purse.

- (i) The patient uses cueing in other specific naming tasks.
- (ii) The patient uses cueing in other treatment tasks, and generalization is established in small steps increasing in difficulty.

When teaching cues it is appropriate to use stimulus material at a level at which the patient's error rate is 50 percent so that the activity provides more opportunities for use of the cueing system.

Criterion response. Responses in LOT are judged as correct or incorrect. Therefore, it is necessary for the clinician to define operationally a correct response, that is, a response that reaches the criterion specified. For example, a conduction aphasic patient may make literal paraphasic errors in a naming task. The clinician, wishing to stress retrieval and not production, may define a criterion response as one that is recognizable as the target response regardless of the presence of literal paraphasias. Later in treatment the criterion response may be increased in difficulty such that only correct productions are accepted. This concept is very important in LOT because it affects whether an increase in the difficulty level is appropriate. It forces clinicians to be very specific about what level of response is acceptable, because ultimately they must decide whether a response will be scored correct or incorrect. This should not be confused with the notion that any response is either "all right" or "all wrong." There are many levels of response difficulty. What it does is define what target response for a given task will meet the criterion and be considered correct and what responses do not meet the criterion and are not included as correct.

Branching. Branching refers to intermediate levels or additional steps to the ones initially outlined in the LOT levels for a patient. It may occur in treatment for two major reasons. If several difficulty levels have been outlined, the clinician may discover that the increases are too difficult. The patient performs at 90 percent on Level 1 but at 20 percent on Level 2, despite repetition of the Level 2 block. Returning to Level 1 is not a good choice and continuing at Level 2 is equally nonproductive. Therefore, the clinician can produce a branch step that is intermediate in difficulty between Levels 1 and 2. Branches should be recorded in the data record and labeled differently from the main levels in the treatment plan. Branching may also occur when several alternatives are available at a particular level in the main program and the clinician knows that the patient requires more repetition than LOT regularly specifies. In working with an aphasic patient in the area of verbal dyspraxia, the clinician may divide a given group of phonemes of equivalent difficulty into three parts, thereby creating three branches. This division would give the aphasic individual considerably more practice than that afforded by a single level without branches. LOT cannot specify with rigid rules when to use branching. The clinician's judgment and the aphasic patient's performance are the important guiding principles. In LOT, each clinician can specify the stimuli presented and the responses obtained. There is an orderly progression in treatment, since advancement in the program is based on the achievement of specified criterion levels. The approach also allows for easy and accurate collection of quantitative data for each patient that can later be analyzed individually and across groups. Of course, such an approach does reduce the flexibility of certain aspects of treatment. However, the advantages of LOT are thought to override this restriction.

Scoring Responses

The aphasic patient's responses should be scored as either correct or incorrect. Whether a patient has made a correct response is determined by whether the response produced meets the criterion set by the clinician. For example, the clinician doing a naming task presents a picture for the patient to name. The patient may produce responses in addition to the target, such as using the word in a sentence. Such additional responses may certainly be encouraged but whether the sentence the patient constructs is correct or not is not relevant in determining the correctness of the response in a naming task. Another patient, asked to identify the word *table* presented auditorily by the clinician, points to the correct picture and says *gable*. The response is correct because the patient did identify the appropriate picture but the clinician should note that the name was still not produced accurately. This information might be used in designing later treatment tasks.

Having response criteria that are flexible for different tasks provides another way of altering the difficulty level of a treatment activity. Target responses can be increased in difficulty independently of the stimuli or cueing support provided by the clinician. In this way the aphasic patient may be able to approach a normal response in several steps, whereas requiring this level initially would have met with failure. LOT does not dictate the steps to be taken in approaching a normal response; this is based on the clinician's judgment and on data gathered during LOT activities. Analyzing a patient's responses in treatment will give the clinician a good basis from which to establish an appropriate hierarchy of increasing difficulty.

The clinician should encourage the patient to respond. Naturally the clinician wants to maximize success, but the patient may need to learn that errors are "not so bad." It is better to make an error in communication than not communicate at all. In addition, the errors will provide clues for the clinician of possible avenues to improve the patient's communication.

Feedback

Feedback to the aphasic patient is very important. It serves to provide knowledge of performance and an objective evaluation of it. Initially, patients may be unable to evaluate their performance, needing to rely on an external evaluation. Eventually, they will want to monitor their own performance as that is closest to a real life situation. Stoicheff (1960) found that when patients received encouraging instructions this positively influenced their performance. Therefore, it is important to encourage the patient. But the clinician must also be honest and stands to lose the patient's trust by saying all is going well when this is obviously not the case.

Positive feedback can be an important source of motivation for the patient. As the old cliché states, "Nothing succeeds like success."

Sequence of Training Activities

Treatment activities are sequenced along two dimensions. One sequence requires increasingly difficult tasks to achieve the content goals established by the clinician. The other organizes the succession of activities within a given treatment session.

The sequence of training activities to achieve a goal, such as improving auditory comprehension of sentences, is guided by a general increase in the difficulty of the task for the patient. Difficulty level can be increased in several ways, as discussed before, and should coincide with the rate of progress in treatment. Briefly, the stimulus material can be more difficult, the cueing can be transferred from the clinician to the patient, or the criterion response can be increased in difficulty. Generally, only one of these aspects is changed at any one time in a treatment activity. However, in a rapidly recovering patient more than one could be increased simultaneously.

Earlier recovery data (Basso, Capitani, and Vignolo, 1979; Hagen, 1973; Henri, 1973; Keenan, 1975) have suggested that recovery in the language modalities occurs in a specific order, with the rank order from earliest to latest being auditory processing, visual processing, oral expression, and graphic expression. This information, when combined with the patient's pattern of language impairment, can help the clinician in decisions about which language modalities to select initially for treatment. If auditory comprehension is impaired it is advisable to train in this modality, since it is difficult to work effectively with a patient who does not understand what is happening in treatment. Graphic expression, because it is usually the most impaired, recovers the least, is less frequently used than the other language modalities, is typically left to later training, or is used less for training than the other modalities. Therefore, it is likely that any LOT training plan will include two or three language modalities, and, of these, auditory processing will be included early if it is impaired and graphic expression will be included later or less intensively. These are, of course, generalities, and individual plans may differ according to the needs of the patient.

Some research data have also indicated that auditory comprehension also shows the greatest amount of recovery (Basso et al., 1979; Henri, 1973). However, more recent data did not confirm this finding (Shewan and Kertesz, 1984). Therefore, the clinician should not be surprised if a patient shows greater recovery in modalities other than auditory processing. Language recovery is an extremely complex phenomenon, the details of which still remain to be discovered.

The sequence of activities within any one treatment session is also an important consideration. The sequence will be individualized for every patient; however, some general guidelines are helpful. Performance in a treatment activity can be influenced by preceding or following events. Knowledge of some general verbal learning principles and concepts, such as proactive and retroactive facilitation and interference, is helpful. Proactive facilitation refers to the general facilitation on performance of an activity prior to training of the target activity. If the learning of B is enhanced by the prior learning of A, proactive facilitation has occurred. One common example is the notion of learning how to learn. Retroactive facilitation refers to the increase in performance of the target activity B, by the subsequent learning of A.

Learn A	Learn B		Recall B	Proactive
	Learn B		Recall B	Control
	Learn B	Learn A	Recall B	Retroactive

Proactive inhibition is analogous to proactive facilitation, only in the latter condition the prior learning of A has the effect of reducing the performance of recalling B, the target activity. Retroactive inhibition is likewise analogous to proactive facilitation except that the subsequent learning of A has a negative influence on the performance of recalling B.

Brookshire (1972) has shown that the aphasic patient's performance on a naming task was influenced by whether the task was preceded by an easy or a difficult naming task. An easy task, when preceded by a difficult one, was performed less well (proactive interference).

A good general rule is to initiate a training session with a task that the clinician believes the patient will perform well. The patient can then be successful initially, and this may provide motivation for the rest of the session. Task difficulty should gradually increase throughout the session, but if perseveration occurs the best procedure is to change the activity. The clinician should always watch the attention span of the patient and terminate a task when the patient is having difficulty attending or is achieving no success. If 20 minutes of the session are to be devoted to auditory comprehension activities, for example, it is preferable to divide this period into two 10-minute blocks rather than to work continuously.

If at all possible training sessions should end on a positive note. This might mean doing a task that the patient generally succeeds at or particularly enjoys.

Clinicians often wonder whether the patient should experience frustration in treatment. Because of the nature of aphasia and because the patient must now function with an impaired system some frustration is bound to occur. If training is error free and the patient never has to work to achieve the goals, the clinician and patient are working below the optimal level for language training. However, the patient should not be continuously frustrated, since this may reduce motivation. It may be very helpful to the patient for the clinician to explain the frustration that occurs. For example, when tasks are increased very slightly in difficulty, the patient may not understand having difficulty with a task that was apparently easy last week. What the patient may not recognize, however, is that the clinician has increased the difficulty, an understanding of which may alleviate the frustration.

Recording Data

Maintaining records for LOT is important for both the clinician and the researcher. Individual goals can be recorded on a LOT Goals form (Fig. 1–6). If a separate form is used for each area within each modality, the successive levels of difficulty and other pertinent information can be recorded across sessions. It has been found to be beneficial to include the stimuli and their method of presentation, what cueing if any is used, the criterion for a correct response, the response method, and any additional responses other than the target response.

MODALITY: _____   CLIENT: _____

AREA: _____   CLINICIAN: _____

GOAL: _____

LOT GOALS

Level	Stimulus	Presentation Method	Cueing Provided	Criterion For Correct Response	Response Method	Additional Responses

Figure 1–6. LOT Goals form to be used to record goals for each area within each modality. It records the level of difficulty, the stimuli and their presentation method, any cueing that is provided, the criterion for a correct response, the response method, and any additional responses. The clinician can use this form to record training both within and across sessions.

The data gathered from each session can be recorded on LOT Data Record forms (Fig. 1–7). It seems most convenient to record each area of each modality on a separate form to preserve continuity across sessions. If training in more than one area in a modality is needed, these forms can be sequenced to assist in the data organization. The session number and date are recorded for identification purposes. To determine how much treatment is provided in different areas, the time spent is recorded in minutes. Clinicians in the recovery study recorded treatment time in this way. Recording the difficulty level of the material allows a cross check with the LOT Goals form. The number of items column will usually contain a 10, since that is the Number of Items in each task or activity. The subject's quantitative performance and any relative qualitative comments are recorded in the data and comments column. Scanning the record for two consecutive blocks of 70 percent or greater achievement at the same level of difficulty signals the clinician to advance to the next level of training as outlined on the LOT Goals form.

If the clinician requires or desires a complete record of a single treatment session on a single record form, the LOT Treatment Plan form can be used (Fig. 1–8). These forms were used in the recovery study by clinicians but are not essential. The same information can be obtained by combining the LOT Goals and Data Record forms for each area trained in a particular session.

Patient-Clinician Interaction

The patient-clinician interaction has been a cornerstone of some treatment approaches. Wepman (1972) considered it a very important aspect of treatment. Many studies have commented on the positive benefits of speech treatment to patients' morale and adjustment to their impairments (Aronson et al., 1956; Blackman and Tureen, 1948).

Engaging in a therapeutic process with an aphasic patient, one is first dealing with a human being, one who has suffered a tremendous loss communicatively and perhaps physically and psychologically. Therefore, treatment involves a psychological dynamic which is not reflected even in a structured language approach like LOT. The clinician interacts with the patient in a caring and considerate manner as with any other treatment approach. The structured language activities occur within the context of a positive communicative and interpersonal environment.

When interacting with aphasic patients it is important to recall some of the literature in which patients told professionals what bothered them about how people interacted with them (Shewan and Cameron, 1984; Skelly, 1975). Clinicians must constantly be aware of these potential problems to help to ease the communication load for aphasic patients. The

MODALITY: _____

AREA: _____

CLIENT: _____

CLINICIAN: _____

LOT DATA RECORD

Session No.	Date	Time Spent (minutes)	Difficulty Level	No. of Items	DATA and COMMENTS

Figure 1-7. LOT Data Record form. This form records identifying information and patient performances for training in an area for the language modality specified.

DATE:_____

SESSION NO: _____

CLIENT: _____

CLINICIAN: _____

LOT TREATMENT PLAN

Modality	Area	Time (minutes)	Level	Stimuli	Responses	Cues

Figure 1-8. LOT Treatment Plan form, which records the relevant treatment information from a single session.

suggestions below are helpful reminders for clinicians and can be given to families, relatives, and friends of the patient as well as to health care professionals (Shewan, undated).

EASING THE COMMUNICATION LOAD WITH THE APHASIC PATIENT

Creating a Good Communication Environment

1. Communicate in a quiet room.
2. Limit the number of people; avoid large groups.
3. Encourage the aphasic patient and stimulate him or her.
4. Recognize and reinforce communication gains.
5. Do not ask the aphasic patient to talk and do something else at the same time.

Be Sensitive to the Aphasic Patient as a Person First, as an Aphasic Individual Second

1. Respect the aphasic person's privacy.
2. Keep the aphasic patient informed about what is happening.
3. Be aware of fatigue.
4. Encourage the aphasic patient to be independent.
5. Keep the aphasic patient occupied.

As a Speaker:

1. Talk slowly.
2. Do not shout.
3. Use appropriate language:
   • short sentences
   • simple sentences
   • familiar words
   • do not bombard the patient with too many questions
4. Stress the important words in sentences.
5. Accompany a message with gestures or repeat if the aphasic person does not undertand.

As a Listener:

1. Listen and do not interrupt.
2. Be patient.

3. Give the aphasic person time to respond.
4. Do not fill in when the aphasic patient cannot find a word.
5. Accept language errors.

Chapter 2

Treatment for Auditory Processing

It is now generally agreed among clinicians and researchers that all aphasic patients demonstrate auditory comprehension problems if tested extensively and with sufficiently difficult tests. These problems vary in their severity and particularly mild ones might not be of sufficient clinical significance to warrant specific treatment. This chapter focuses on those problems sufficiently severe to interfere with an aphasic patient's ability to function in our auditory world in general, in a particular profession, or in both.

Various types of auditory processing deficits occur in the aphasic population. Most prominent is that of an impairment in the comprehension of meaningful language, or auditory comprehension, which will be emphasized here. However, auditory agnosia, pure word deafness, and auditory imperception will be discussed briefly since they do occur in aphasia, although rarely.

TYPES OF AUDITORY PROCESSING DEFICITS

Some types of auditory processing deficits are briefly reviewed here. For a more extensive description, the reader is referred to Shewan (1982).

Auditory Comprehension Impairment

Comprehension of spoken language requires processing the linguistic input (word, sentence, or discourse) phonologically, semantically, and syntactically. Independent processing in each of these components as well as interactive processing among them are required in normal comprehension. It is with this processing that most aphasic individuals have difficulty. Although they can hear and perceive speech, they have difficulty understanding it.

Comprehension of linguistic messages is related to certain suprasegmental phonological parameters such as stress, intonation, and juncture in addition to the accurate perception of speech. Although speech discrimination problems do occur in aphasia, they are generally not the prime factor interfering with comprehension. The perception of stress as a phonemic cue, as in "récord" versus "récord," seems to be maintained in aphasic adults (Blumstein and Goodglass, 1972). Stress as a suprasegmental cue in sentences, however, can influence comprehension performance (Goodglass, 1975, 1976; Kellar, 1978; Pashek and Brookshire, 1980). Boller and Green (1972) and Green and Boller (1974) found that patients with severe comprehension problems matched questions, statements, and commands with appropriate response categories, suggesting they were obtaining some information from intonation contour, even though their responses were not correct. Although the cues provided by intonation contour may be redundant for normal adults, they may be used by some aphasic patients.

Most frequently the clinician is concerned with semantic and syntactic components as they influence the auditory comprehension of aphasic individuals. They comprehend common, frequently occurring material better than uncommon, rare, unfamiliar material. An aphasic patient may correctly identify "chair" but not "divan," since the former word is more frequently occurring in English. Frequency of occurrence has its influence whether the words occur separately or whether they are embedded in a sentence context. When material becomes more complex, such as with longer length or more complex syntactic construction, aphasic subjects have more difficulty comprehending it. For example, Shewan (1979) demonstrated these effects using the Auditory Comprehension Test for Sentences (ACTS). Some aphasic subjects could comprehend a sentence like "The girl is reading a book" but not "The little old lady stands on the bank beside the river," since the syllable length of the latter sentence is more than twice that of the former—although the vocabulary difficulty and syntactic complexity of the two sentences are comparable. Other aphasic patients often had difficulty comprehending "The dogs are not chased by cats," although they comprehended "The dogs are chasing the cats." The syntactic construction of the first sentence, reversible and negative-passive, makes it more complex than the second sentence, which is simple, active, affirmative, and declarative. Note that the two sentences are comparable for length and vocabulary difficulty.

Problems in comprehension may also arise if the situational context minimizes the availability of other cues, nonlinguistic cues, since these are present in many communication situations and may be used to aid in understanding. Presentation method of the material can influence comprehension; slowing the rate of speech and/or inserting pauses at strategic points facilitates comprehension for some patients. Likewise, response variables can influence comprehension performance. The number and type of response choices as well as the scoring system used, for example, whether completeness and latency are scored as well as accuracy, will affect judgments about comprehension. Emotional content and familiarity of content can both be facilitating to auditory comprehension in aphasic patients. The point to be made is that whether a given linguistic message is understood by an aphasic patient depends not only on the linguistic content of that message but also on other variables, such as context and so on.

Auditory Imperception

This term used currently to refer to a type of aphasia (Jenkins et al., 1975) describes the phenomenon in which an aphasic patient seems to fade in and out in the understanding of spoken language. Analogous to a camera shutter, the patient can understand when the shutter is open but not when it is closed. These periods of imperception vary in duration from only a few seconds to several minutes (Brookshire, 1978). Patients with auditory imperception present other language deficits as well, often fluent speech characterized by jargon. These patients often appear confused and anxious in verbal communication situations since they cannot understand what is transpiring. They may understand longer messages but miss shorter ones because of their ability to integrate separate segments of the longer command.

Jenkins and co-workers (1975) reported that almost half the aphasic patients of this type had bilateral brain damage, Schuell and associates (1964) advocated improving speech perception and discrimination, which would eventually lead to being able to assign meaning to auditory stimuli. Perhaps this would help those in whom difficulty with aspects of speech perception predominated, as described by Jenkins and co-workers (1975). However, with other patients whose primary problems were deriving meaning from what was said, Schuell's approach would not appear appropriate.

Auditory imperception formed the basis of the problems in sensory (acoustic-agnostic) aphasia, as described by Luria (1980). Damage to the cortical division of the auditory analyzer system interfered with the analysis and synthesis of speech sounds, which resulted in a problem of phonemic hearing that, in turn, manifested itself in both receptive and expressive language tasks. This problem of phonemic hearing disturbed phonemic discrimination and also related to the conceptual impairment in aphasia, since the word meaning system was based on the phonemic structure of speech.

Pure Word Deafness

Pure word deafness refers to a patient's inability to understand spoken language in the face of other language modalities being spared. Although word deafness is rarely pure and may be associated with aphasia (Gazzaniga, Glass, Sarno, and Posner, 1973; Marshall and Stevenson, 1977), it is striking in its relatively profound impairment in interpreting auditory verbal stimuli. The patient cannot understand single words and has difficulty with repetition and writing to dictation owing to the auditory presentation of the stimuli. Temporal resolution problems (Albert and Baer, 1974) and prephonetic auditory perceptual problems (Saffran, Marin, and Yeni-Komshian, 1976) have both been used as explanations of this syndrome.

Auditory Agnosia

Auditory agnosia is a term that has been used to describe two syndromes. In its restricted definition, auditory nonverbal agnosia, it refers to the inability to recognize nonverbal auditory stimuli, such as environmental sounds, with the preservation of auditory comprehension. Auditory nonverbal agnosia may occur with other deficits, often pure word deafness. Albert, Sparks, Von Stockert, and Sax (1972) noted impaired auditory localization, left-sided neglect, and impaired perception of pitch, loudness, rhythm, and time in their patient with auditory agnosia. A more extensive condition, in which inability to recognize both nonverbal and verbal stimuli are present, has been referred to as "auditory verbal agnosia" or "pure word deafness" (Benson, 1979).

GENERAL GUIDELINES FOR AUDITORY PROCESSING TREATMENT

The treatment guidelines for auditory processing deficits have been divided into two major categories, those pertaining to auditory perceptual deficits and those encompassing auditory comprehension deficits. This division reflects differences in the stimuli involved in the category (e.g., environmental sounds versus short sentences), the auditory processes focused on (e.g., awareness versus comprehension), or both. For most aphasic patients, treatment will focus on comprehension deficits. However, in some aphasic patients, the auditory problem is so severe that comprehension is not possible (Boller and Green, 1972). For these patients, treatment would begin with perceptual activities, such as discriminating among auditory stimuli, to engage them in processing auditory stimuli, with the goal of making the transition to comprehending speech stimuli as soon as possible. As a general rule, perceptual tasks are used only when needed and the focus of therapy is to have the patient understand meaningful language.

Each of the two major categories has been subdivided into more specific areas, with the intention of segmenting the "auditory processing pie" into mutually exclusive areas from which clinicians can select one or more for training. The auditory perceptual category has been divided into three areas: awareness of auditory stimuli, recognition of auditory stimuli, and monitoring speech. The division was important so that each therapy activity could be classified appropriately and so that no activity would fall into more than one area. This also allows for replication of the method across clinicians and for consistent and reliable data collection. The auditory comprehension category is composed of six areas: comprehension of single units, comprehension of short series, comprehension of short meaningful linguistic units, comprehension of sentences, comprehension of paragraphs, and comprehension of narratives and discourse. Which areas are selected during the course of treatment is determined by the client's performance on standardized test batteries and by supplementary testing if necessary. Therefore, the areas treated will depend on the nature of the patient's auditory processing problems and level of functioning.

Within each category, where possible, the areas have been arranged according to difficulty. For example, all other things being equal, it is generally more difficult to comprehend sentences than single words. This does not mean that comprehending sentences would be an area selected only after all treatment had been completed with single words. Rather, the most frequent situation would be both areas being treated simultaneously but at different levels within each area. For example, the patient might be identifying moderately difficult single words and comprehending very short simple sentences. Therefore, in any given session, activities for auditory processing might occur in several areas, the specific areas and levels within them being dictated by the nature and the degree of the patient's problem.

Within sessions and across sessions, as the patient is able to successfully accomplish each level in a hierarchy, its difficulty is increased, with the result that the patient progresses through a series of tasks, which gradually increase in difficulty. Within each area, as much detailed information as possible is provided regarding a hierarchy of difficulty for materials. The hierarchies have been based on the current neurolinguistic, neuropsychological, psycholinguistic, and aphasia literature available, which provides information about auditory processing of aphasic patients—what tasks are easy, what tasks are difficult, and what variables influence performance. Of course, the information is not complete and where gaps exist, we have deferred to processing information available from normal adults to create task hierarchies. Only additional research will reveal whether this is an appropriate model; at present, it is one possibility.

The hierarchies will not hold true for every aphasic patient, and consequently, finding the patient's particular pattern is important through testing or using the baselining techniques described earlier. Where sufficient data were not available from which to organize hierarchies of difficulty, the hierarchies are only suggestive and the individual's baseline performance will determine the appropriate difficulty levels.

An aphasic patient's auditory performance depends on the stimuli to be processed, but the linguistic message is not the only variable determining a response. The situational context, extralinguistic variables, response variables, and presentation variables can also influence success or failure. Therefore, these variables are manipulated as well as the stimulus variables to increase the task difficulty. For example, the aphasic patient's task is to comprehend simple phrases and to select the appropriate picture that matches the phrase. At first, the clinician stresses the crucial words, repeats the stimulus twice, and has the patient select from two options. The next stage might be to increase the number of options from which to select, to omit the repetition, or to remove the exaggerated stress. Therefore, the clinician has three options and which one is chosen will depend on the individual patient. Each of these options could be applied in turn to increase the difficulty of the task three levels, even though the difficulty of the stimuli do not increase. Of course, the actual stimulus phrases change so that the patient is not learning specific stimuli but rather learning to process stimuli of a given difficulty. The goal is to increase the difficulty of the stimuli to be comprehended and to have the patient rely less on the clinician providing additional cues or prompts in order to be successful. Initially, the clinician cues the patient and tries to teach a strategy. For example, extra stress on words is a cue used, while the clinician tells the patient to listen for the stressed words as they are the important cues to meaning. Gradually, the cues are reduced and the patient uses the strategy on his own. Subsequently, the stimuli selected are more complex with a readjustment in cues and strategies as necessary.

Treatment would continue in auditory processing until the patient had "plateaued" or until auditory processing skills had recovered. The next two sections will provide clinicians with guidelines for establishing treatment hierarchies in their aphasic patients.

GUIDELINES FOR AUDITORY PERCEPTUAL PROCESSING DEFICITS

Treatment using auditory perceptual tasks is not meant to be the focus for auditory processing, but some aphasic individuals are not able to perform the comprehension tasks. They may demonstrate auditory perceptual problems that involve discrimination, recognition, temporal ordering, or a combination of these. The deficits may be found using verbal or nonverbal material. They are not exclusive to patients with Wernicke's aphasia but extend to other aphasic groups as well. Nor do they completely explain auditory comprehension problems in aphasic patients. Perceptual problems are associated with auditory comprehension problems in some aphasic patients; they are not associated in others, since some pass auditory comprehension tests and fail discrimination tests (Carpenter and Rutherford, 1973).

The materials are included here for two kinds of situations. If an aphasic patient cannot succeed with any comprehension tasks, using perceptual tasks may be helpful. In this way, activities could be used as precursors to later comprehension tasks. Transferring to comprehension from awareness or recognition tasks is recommended as soon as possible. Aphasic patients who have severe auditory comprehension problems may not be able to comprehend the linguistic meaning of auditory materials, although they may be able to process them at a different level, such as discrimination. Using perceptual analytical tasks may facilitate the transition to comprehending auditory stimuli.

To summarize, do not focus on auditory perceptual tasks if the aphasic patient can succeed with comprehension tasks. Focus on comprehension with these patients. If auditory perceptual problems are interfering with auditory comprehension, training with perceptual tasks may be used to have the patient tune into the auditory modality and/or to ready the mechanism for comprehension activities. Unfortunately, evidence that the training will have this effect does not exist.

The first two areas deal with the processes of awareness and recognition. The latter process involves a comparison of the stimulus to some memory trace in the brain to determine if they match. Therefore, correspondence tasks are involved. The last area, monitoring, requires the added process of judging whether a stimulus is correct; that is, does it match patterns standard for the language? The monitoring process is particularly important for Wernicke's aphasic patients to make them attend to whether their verbal output is appropriate or accurate, or both.

Area 1: Awareness of Auditory Stimuli

1. Awareness of Nonspeech Stimuli

Stimuli. The stimuli here can be environmental sounds or music. One is not deemed more difficult than another.

Description. Activities are designed to have the aphasic patient attend to auditory stimuli. The task is to respond differentially when the auditory stimuli are presented.

Example. The aphasic individual raises a hand when music is present on a tape recording.

2. Awareness of Speech Stimuli

Stimuli. Speech stimuli from familiar speakers, unfamiliar speakers, or from a foreign language are used. The stimuli most likely to arouse the aphasic patient are familiar speakers, because of their familiarity, or foreign language stimuli, because of their novelty.

Description. The activities are designed to make the patient aware of speech stimuli. The patient does not have to recognize the stimuli but has to respond differentially to speech versus nonspeech stimuli.

Example. The patient points to a picutre of a person when a voice is heard and to a picture of a musical instrument when music is heard.

Area 2: Recognition of Auditory Stimuli

1. Recognition of Nonspeech Stimuli

Stimuli. The stimuli can be environmental sounds, music, or rhythmical patterns.

Description. Activities are for the purpose of associating particular auditory stimuli with appropriate referents in the environment.

Example. The patient matches environmental sounds, such as a telephone ringing, to the appropriate environmental referent, a real telephone or a photograph of one.

2. Recognition of Speech Stimuli

Stimuli. The stimuli consist of familiar and unfamiliar speakers using normal English, speakers using semantic jargon, or speakers using a foreign language.

Description. The goal is to have the aphasic patient recognize what is English versus other linguistic stimuli that are not linguistically meaningful to him or her. The patient does not have to comprehend the stimuli, however.

Example. The patient listens to a tape recording and indicates if it sounds "okay." The recording will randomly present English stimuli versus Spanish stimuli.

3.   Recognition of Communicative Intent of a Message

Stimuli. These stimuli, used by Green and Boller (1974), are listed in a hierarchy from least to most difficult.

Easy	Command
↓	Yes-no question
Difficult	Information question

Description. Activities in this segment are designed to encourage the aphasic patient to attend to cues such as intonation and stress patterns, which will indicate the semantic intent of the speaker, whether giving directions or asking a particular kind of question.

Example. On hearing a command, the aphasic patient responds with a gesture thereby indicating recognition that it is necessary to do something. When presented with a wh question, the patient gives some type of verbal response other than "yes" or "no" to indicate he or she recognizes that some type of information is required. It is important to remember that the correct gesture or the correct information are not required for success in this area; the response, however, need only be appropriate; that is, a gesture is appropriate to a command but not to a wh question.

Area 3: Monitoring Speech

Stimuli. The stimuli, which are rank ordered, can be any units of speech from single words to conversation.

Easy	Single Words
	Phrases
↓	Sentences
Difficult	Conversation

Description. Activities are designed that demonstrate whether the aphasic patient monitors the accuracy and/or meaningfulness of speech stimuli. These may be his or her own productions or those of the clinician or family. These activities are precursors to self-correction in the patient who makes errors but does not appear to be aware of them. Wernicke's aphasic patients are the group that most frequently fail to monitor their speech.

Example. The aphasic patient is describing pictures using short phrases, such as "in the sink," "on the box," and so forth. The clinician provides the correct answer. The patient listens to the recorded answer and judges whether it matches the clinician's.

GUIDELINES FOR AUDITORY COMPREHENSION DEFICITS

For patients with deficits in this category, treatment can be provided in one or more of the following six areas. As mentioned in the previous chapter, which area or areas are selected and at what level training begins is determined by a thorough evaluation of auditory comprehension. Information can come from standardized tests and from clinician-generated tests. For example, on the Boston Diagnostic Aphasia Examination (BDAE) (Goodglass and Kaplan, 1972), the patient had difficulty with understanding commands. The clinician might then choose to work on the area "Comprehension of Sentences," but since the stimuli of the BDAE are all commands, he or she would need to investigate further which sentence types and the parameters of these types the patient can and cannot understand. The rank order of difficulty of various sentence types has been listed. This order was based on studies that required aphasic subjects to comprehend single sentences. Since each aphasic patient is unique, it would be beneficial to sample sentences at several levels to determine at what point the patient starts to have difficulty. Recall that stimulus material should be selected at a level where the patient achieves a rate of 50 to 70 percent correct. This level provides that the patient will make some errors and, therefore, has an opportunity to apply the cues or strategies being taught. If the material is too easy, the patient is not challenged to achieve a higher goal. Criterion for advancing to a higher level has frequently been selected as achievement of 70 percent or more on two consecutive stimulus sets, each containing 10 homogeneous stimuli. Depending on the patient, this can be adjusted to 80 percent or 90 percent. However, the idea is not to restrain the patient from progressing because he or she makes the odd error.

The therapy task can be made more difficult by increasing the level of the stimuli (based on the hierarchies outlined), by altering presentation variables, by requiring a more complex response, by providing less context, or by altering extralinguistic variables. In general, it is recommended that only one variable at a time be altered to increase the task difficulty. In this way, the clinician knows why a particular task was easier or more difficult than the previous one. If a client can progress faster than this, and this becomes evident in the first few treatment sessions, then the size of the steps between difficulty levels can and should be increased. The client's performance signals the clinician when to advance and by how much.

Each area is organized so that the stimuli appropriate for that level are indicated. Unless specified otherwise, they are listed in rank order from easiest to most difficult. Variables that affect performance with these stimuli and are therefore important to control are listed. A description of the types of activities that would be appropriate for each area are described, along with an example provided. Additional examples of clinical activities for each area are described in Chapter 3 of this book.

Area 4: Comprehension of Single Units

Stimuli.   In general, this area deals with the comprehension of single words. The stimulus words can be organized into difficulty levels using a variety of parameters. The following hierarchies show the differences according to semantic categories (Goodglass, Klein, Carey, and Jones, 1966).

	Broca's	Wernicke's	Anomic
Easy	Body parts	Body parts	Body parts
	Actions	Actions	Objects
	Objects	Objects	Actions
	Numbers	Numbers	Numbers
	Colors	Letters	Colors
	Letters	Colors	Letters
Difficult	Geometric forms	Forms	Forms

Frequency of occurrence of words has been shown to be directly related to comprehension. As frequency of occurrence increases, so does the likelihood that a given word will be comprehended accurately. Therefore, it is important to establish at what level of difficulty a patient is functioning. Several sources are listed that rank order words in English. These sources can be used in creating hierarchies of difficulty, by gradually decreasing word frequency:

Carroll, J. B., Davies, P., and Richman, B. (1971). *The American Heritage word frequency book.* Boston: Houghton-Mifflin Co.
Griffith, J., and Miner, L. E. (1973). *The language master articulation and therapy program.* Chicago: Bell & Howell.
Kuçera, H., and Francis, W. N. (1967). *Computational analysis of present day English.* Providence, RI: Brown University Press.
Thorndike, H. L., and Lorge, I (1944). *The teacher's word book of 30,000 words.* New York: Columbia University.

Wepman, J. M., and Jones, L. V. (1966). *A spoken word count.* Chicago: Language Research Associates, Inc.

The evidence on whether grammatical form class is important to control is conflicting. Grammatical classes have not been systematically compared and function words have usually been studied in the context of sentence material (Parisi and Pizzamiglio, 1970). In this context, function words are more difficult to comprehend than content words (Caramazza, Zurif, and Gardner, 1978). Goodglass, Gleason, and Hyde (1970) provide some information about prepositions. Shewan (1976a), using the ACTS sentence comprehension test, did not find a greater proportion of errors for any one grammatical form class (noun, verb, adjective, pronoun) than was expected by chance. The best approach would appear to include several grammatical form classes as part of a baseline measure to determine any potential differences for a particular patient.

Description. The purpose of activities in this area is to improve the aphasic patient's ability to understand single units such as common words, colors, and so on. These stimuli are presented auditorily and the patient generally points to an appropriate picture or object or demonstrates an appropriate action.

Example. The aphasic patient points to the appropriate picture corresponding to the prepositions "in" and "under."

Area 5: Comprehension of Short Series

Stimuli. This area encompasses processing short series of stimuli such as numbers, phonemes, letters, or words. Although the aphasic patient is not expected to abstract a relationship among the stimuli, assumedly items in the same series category will be more easily processed than several items from different categories.

In general, series of numbers, since they are highly familiar, are easier to process than phoneme or letter series. The difficulty of word series will depend on those variables discussed in Area 1, such as word frequency and semantic categories. There may be individual exceptions to the hierarchy, which the clinician should note. The information from the semantic category hierarchies for Area 4 can be used as a basis for a task hierarchy, or baseline data can be used to establish one.

Easy	Word series
↓	Number series
	Phoneme series
Difficult	Letter series

Immediate or short-term memory or both are involved in these tasks. Repetition of an item in the series will make it easier, all other things being equal.

Longer series will be more difficult than shorter ones. In word series, words that cluster into the same category may be easier than unrelated word series (Tillman and Gerstman, 1977).

Description. These activities are designed to facilitate aphasic patients' processing of longer series. They stress memory capabilities as well as auditory processing. They can serve as a bridge or as an alternative to processing shorter meaningful linguistic units discussed in Area 3. That the items do not form a syntactic unit forces the patient to attend to each member by itself. For the aphasic patient progress from processing single units to series can be facilitated by focusing on rehearsal strategies, such as chunking or repetition. Although aphasic patients do have difficulty using chunking strategies, some can take advantage of them. Repeating the series subvocally may also help, as might encouraging the patient to use a visual imagery strategy. These are all important to use as support, which can then gradually be incorporated by the aphasic patient to successfully perform these tasks.

Example. The clinician presents a three-number series auditorily and the aphasic patient points to the correct series, from a choice of two.

Area 6: Comprehension of Short Meaningful Linguistic Units

Stimuli. The difference between this area and the previous one is that the stimuli are related into syntactic units, either as linguistic constituents or as short complete sentences. The first stimulus set is not listed in a hierarchy, since no experimental data were available to support rank ordering them. The second stimulus set is rank ordered. As combinations of units found in English, each contains two or three content items:

Adjective + Noun
Adjective + Pronoun
Preposition + Noun
Preposition + Pronoun
Noun + Verb
Pronoun + Verb

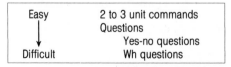

Easy	2 to 3 unit commands
	Questions
↓	Yes-no questions
Difficult	Wh questions

Several stimulus variables are important to control in these units. As for the previous areas, using frequently occurring words within the units will make comprehension easier, as will dealing with highly familiar topics.

For the complete grammatical units, controlling sentence type is also important. All other things being equal, commands and yes-no questions are easier to comprehend than wh questions. The short length and limited content units put these constructions into this area rather than Area 7.

Description. Activities in this area are designed to improve the aphasic patient's ability to understand simple, short, meaningful combinations of lexical items. They are further designed to have the aphasic patient attend to more than one item in a speaker's verbalization.

Example. The aphasic patient is asked to carry out simple commands such as "Make a fist" or "Close your eyes." Initially, these types of activities could be presented auditorily with an accompanying gesture from the clinician. As the patient progressed, the gesture would be faded out. Be sure with this type of gestural task to screen for limb apraxia and oral apraxia.

Area 7: Comprehension of Sentences

Stimuli. The stimuli for treatment in this area consist of sentences of various types. Within each type, the sentences can be made easier or more difficult by altering several parameters, such as length, grammatical contrasts, truth value, and so on. The first hierarchy of sentences, representing a compilation of several authors' work, is organized from easy to difficult (Table 2–1) (Caramazza and Zurif, 1978; Levy and Taylor, 1968; Parisi and Pizzamiglio, 1970; Shewan and Canter, 1971).

An addition within this hierarchy is appropriate if reaction time rather than accuracy of response is considered. False simple active affirmative declarative (SAAD) sentences and false reversible passives are reacted to more quickly than true SAAD and true reversible passives (Brookshire and Nicholas, 1980).

A second addition is that compound sentences conjoined with "and" are easier than center-embedded sentences (Goodglass et al., 1979).

The next hierarchy consists of seven types of wh questions listed in order of difficulty according to Gallagher and Guilford's findings (1977). The example is from their work. The questions are asked about a test picture in which a woman is washing dishes at a kitchen sink. She is holding a dinner plate.

Easy	Type	Question
	What—do	What is she doing?
	How many	How many are there?
	Who	Who is washing?
	What—verb	What is she washing?
	What kind	What size is it?
	Where	Where is she washing?
Difficult	When	When is she washing?

Table 2-1. Hierarchy of Difficulty for Sentence Types from Easy to Difficult

Sentence Type

Simple Active Affirmative Declarative (SAAD)
 E.g., The dog is chasing the cat.
 Negative
 E.g., The dog is not chasing the cat.
 Passive
 A. Nonreversible
     E.g., The ball is being caught by the dog.
 B. Reversible
     E.g., The cat is being chased by the dog.
 Negative-passive
 E.g., The cat is not being chased by the dog.
 Center-embedded
 A. Nonreversible
     E.g., The cat that the dog is chasing is meowing.
 B. Reversible
     E.g., The cat that the dog is chasing is black.

Easy → Difficult (indicated by downward arrow at left of table)

Sentences that follow an order of mention strategy are more accurately comprehended than those that do not (Ansell and Flowers, 1980).

The literature in aphasia has also contained data that indicate that some grammatical contrasts are easier for aphasic patients than are others. The following grammatical contrasts are rank ordered according to difficulty as found in three studies (Table 2–2) (Lesser, 1974, 1978; Parisi and Pizzamiglio, 1970; Pierce, 1979).

Description. The activities in this area are designed to improve the aphasic patient's ability to comprehend sentences. Simple active affirmative sentences are generally easier to understand than other types. However, it is important to remember that any given type of sentence can be made more difficult by increasing its length, including particular grammatical contrasts, or using less common vocabulary. These variables can be used by the clinician to expand the hierarchies as needed.

Example. A sentence is presented auditorily to the aphasic patient who then selects the correct picture, from among four, which matches the sentence heard.

Area 8: Comprehension of Paragraphs

Stimuli. The stimuli in this area consist of longer units of related material. Paragraph comprehension requires the aphasic patient to understand more material and also to relate that material together. Therefore, paragraph comprehension differs from individual sentence materials in that generally there is more material to process, both longer in syllable length and greater in amount of content. The material can vary in complex-

Table 2–2.   Comparison of Grammatical Contrasts as Rank Ordered in Three Studies

			Pierce (1979)	
Grammatical Contrast	Lesser (1974)	Parisi and Pizzamiglio (1970)	NF–HAC*	COMBINED†
Word Order				
Reversible active	1‡	4		
Direct–indirect object	4	1	5	4
From-to	7	11		
Reversible passive	2	2	4	3
Subordinate clause (relative clause)	5	8.5		
Verb tense				
Present-past	7	3	3, 1	5, 2
Present-future	3	5	2	1
Singular-plural				
Possessive pronoun	10	8.5		
Noun (± verb)	13	16		
Negative-affirmative				
Is-isn't	19.5	15	6	6
Pronoun				
Reflexive-nonreflexive	16.5	6		
Gender				
Male-female	19.5	14		
Locative prepositions				
"Difficult"				
To-from	10	7		
Behind-beside	10	10		
Beside-between	7	12		
"Easy"				
Behind-in front of	13	17		
On-under	13	13		
Near-away from	16.5	20		
In-out of	18	19		
Up-down	15	18		

*NF-HAC = Nonfluent high auditory comprehension group.
†COMBINED = Combined groups of nonfluent low auditory comprehension, fluent high auditory comprehension, and fluent low auditory comprehension.
‡1, The most difficult item; 20, the easiest item.

ity by altering the syntactic complexity of the sentences and by varying the aphasic patient's familiarity or interest in the material (Shewan, 1982; tachowiak, Huber, Pöeck, and Kerschensteiner, 1977).

A definite hierarchy is difficult to establish because it is based on several parameters, all of which can be varied independently. The relevant parameters are listed and the overall difficulty of a paragraph can be determined by rating the difficulty level of each one and arriving at an overall value. Although this is not a totally objective procedure, it is based on some quantitative evaluation rather than a global subjective judgment. The drawback is that in a cumulative complexity paradigm, all variables are assumed to increase complexity in an additive manner, which may not reflect reality.

> **Variables to Control**
> Length of sentences
> Syntactic complexity of sentences
> Vocabulary difficulty in paragraph
> Degree of topic familiarity
> Degree of patient interest in topic
> Amount of content (facts)
> Cohesion among sentence units

Description. Paragraph comprehension tasks are designed to have the aphasic patient understand longer material and to abstract a general idea from the whole. Therefore, the patient is required not only to process and to recall factual material but also to relate the factual material together. Testing can be varied to focus on ability to recall facts or to abstract inferences.

Example. The aphasic patient answers several yes-no questions following a paragraph read to him or her. The paragraph was 60 words in length and contained vocabulary at a third to fourth grade level.

Area 9: Comprehension of Narratives and Discourse

Stimuli. Stimuli in this area differ from the previous one in their format, length, and style. Narratives can vary in length from the short reports of newscast items to an hour lecture or talk on a particular topic. A variety of radio programs use a narrative format by reviewing consumer products, relating biographical material, describing travel, and so forth. Short stories or complete books are also available in audio form. The other kind of stimulus is discourse, often in the form of conversation. Conversation occurs frequently in most people's lives and is important for aphasic patients as a vehicle for everyday interaction. Comprehending narratives and conversation depends to a large extent on the sentence subcomponents comprising them. Because of this, it is difficult to establish a set hierarchy. However, the variables outlined in Area 8 can be considered in constructing or selecting stimulus items.

Variable to Control
Degree of shared information with speaker

Description. Activities are designed to have the aphasic patient comprehend materials that are likely to be encountered in everyday life. The materials often require the patient to retain a series of events, to interact with the speaker, or both. Although the last area listed in auditory comprehension and often containing the most complex stimuli, these activities could be altered to include very simple conversational activities that would be no more difficult than comprehending simple sentences or questions. They have been included in this area to reflect that they are generally more advanced. This is a good example of the previously mentioned concept that, although the areas were selected to represent increasing complexity, a similar degree of complexity can overlap across areas.

Example. The aphasic patient listens to a short radio program, perhaps 5 minutes, and selects from a list provided by the clinician the major ideas that were presented.

Chapter 3

Materials for Auditory Processing

AUDITORY PERCEPTUAL DEFICITS

Area 1: Awareness of Auditory Stimuli

Beginning Levels

Level 1

Stimuli. Tape recorded environmental sounds and music

Procedure. Patient raises a hand when the environmental sound or music is presented on the tape and lowers it when the sound is terminated.

Set A

1. piano
2. whistle blowing
3. door slamming
4. telephone ring
5. alarm clock
6. fire alarm
7. liquid being poured
8. hammering
9. vacuum cleaner
10. door bell

Level 2

Stimuli. Tape recorded human or animal sounds

Procedure. Patient raises a hand when the voiced stimulus is presented on the tape and lowers it when the sound is terminated.

Set A

1. baby's crying
2. laughter
3. humming
4. duck quacking
5. cat meowing
6. children singing
7. man's voice
8. woman's voice
9. young child's voice
10. dog barking

Level 3

Stimuli. A combination of tape recorded environmental sounds and music and voiced productions

Procedure. Patient raises a hand only when a voiced production is presented and keeps it lowered during presentation of environmental sounds.

Set A	Set B
1. piano	1. baby's crying
2. harp	2. laughter
3. door slamming	3. humming
4. telephone ring	4. trumpet
5. alarm clock	5. guitar
6. fire alarm	6. children singing
7. liquid being poured	7. man's voice
8. hammering	8. woman's voice
9. vacuum cleaner	9. young child's voice
10. door bell	10. drums

Area 2: Recognition of Auditory Stimuli

Beginning Levels

Level 1

Stimuli. Tape recorded environmental sounds and music. Pictured items to correspond to the environmental sounds and music.

Procedure. The environmental sound or music is presented along with two pictured stimuli. The patient points to the appropriate picture (underlined in Set A).

Set A

1.	telephone ring	car horn
2.	airplane	door bell
3.	typewriter	whistle blowing
4.	liquid being poured	car starting
5.	cash register	vacuum cleaner
6.	hammering	motorcycle
7.	piano	train
8.	door slamming	toilet flushing
9.	person running	alarm clock
10.	fire alarm	traffic noises

Level 2

Stimuli. Tape recorded samples of English and other linguistic stimuli that are not normally linguistically meaningful to the patient. For example, samples of speech spoken in French can be alternated with English stimuli.

Procedure. The patient raises a hand when the English stimuli are presented. Opportunities for 10 responses should be provided before advancing to the next level.

Level 3

Stimuli. Commands, yes-no questions

Procedure. Commands and yes-no questions are randomly presented auditorily to the patient. The patient responds with a gesture to indicate recognition of a command and with "yes" or "no" to indicate recognition of a question. The correct gesture or yes-no response is not required for success.

Set A

1. Close your eyes.
2. Raise your hand.
3. Are you a nurse?
4. Point to the door.
5. Am I your mother?
6. Take off your glasses.
7. Comb your hair.
8. Is this a restaurant?
9. Are you wearing pajamas?
10. Is the door open?

Set B

1. Do dogs bark?
2. Is the sun hot?
3. Point to your nose.
4. Open your mouth.
5. Pick up the pen.
6. Is today Sunday?
7. Are you sitting down?
8. Show me your ring.
9. Do you drink coffee?
10. Knock on the table.

Additional Levels

Additional levels may be developed by introducing information questions. When presented with a wh question, the patient is required to give some verbal response other than "yes" or "no" indicating recognition that some type of information is required.

Area 3: Monitoring Speech

Intermediate Levels

Level 1

Procedure. The clinician auditorily presents a subject-verb-object utterance in response to an action picture. Some of the sentences are grammatically correct and some are not. The patient is required to determine whether or not a given utterance is grammatically correct.

Level 2

Stimuli. Action pictures

Procedure. The patient is required to formulate a subect-verb-object utterance following presentation of an action picture. This response is tape recorded and played back. The patient is required to judge whether or not the utterance is grammatically correct.

Level 3

Stimuli. Action pictures

Procedure. The patient is required to formulate a subject-verb-object utterance following presentation of an action picture. She or he is required immediately to judge whether or not the response is grammatically correct.

Additional Levels

Additional levels may be developed by requiring the patient to monitor the productions for phonemic accuracy, sentence completeness, and content appropriateness.

AUDITORY COMPREHENSION DEFICITS

Area 4: Comprehension of Single Units

Beginning Levels

Level 1

Stimuli. Pictured nouns, unrelated series; grades 1 and 2 vocabulary; monosyllabic nouns

Set A	Set B
1. bed	1. egg
2. dog	2. watch
3. boat	3. salt
4. tree	4. rose
5. dress	5. cup
6. book	6. box
7. car	7. house
8. suit	8. sky
9. glass	9. milk
10. coat	10. wife

Procedure. The following sets of three pictured nouns are placed in front of the patient. The clinician auditorily presents the underlined word and the patient points to the appropriate picture. Possible sources of pictured stimuli for this and subsequent levels and areas are included in the list at the end of this chapter.

Set A

1.	<u>bed</u>	cup	tree
2.	watch	dress	<u>dog</u>
3.	<u>boat</u>	cup	house
4.	<u>tree</u>	egg	wife
5.	sky	<u>dress</u>	box
6.	rose	milk	<u>book</u>
7.	glass	egg	<u>car</u>
8.	<u>suit</u>	bed	egg
9.	dog	<u>glass</u>	dress
10.	salt	<u>coat</u>	box

Set B

1. egg	<u>bed</u>	suit
2. <u>watch</u>	car	milk
3. book	wife	<u>salt</u>
4. rose	<u>box</u>	house
5. tree	<u>cup</u>	dress
6. <u>box</u>	glass	egg
7. house	book	<u>dress</u>
8. <u>sky</u>	dog	coat
9. bed	milk	<u>dress</u>
10. <u>wife</u>	rose	cup

Level 2

Stimuli. Pictured nouns, related series, grades 1 and 2 vocabulary; monosyllabic words

Set A	Set B
1. bed	1. egg
2. dog	2. watch
3. boat	3. salt
4. tree	4. rose
5. dress	5. cup
6. book	6. box
7. car	7. house
8. suit	8. sky
9. glass	9. milk
10. coat	10. wife

Procedure. The following sets of three pictured nouns are placed in front of the patient. The clinician auditorily presents the underlined word and the patient points to the appropriate picture.

Set A

1. chair	<u>bed</u>	sofa
2. <u>dog</u>	cat	horse
3. car	plane	<u>boat</u>
4. leaf	rose	<u>tree</u>
5. skirt	coat	<u>dress</u>
6. magazine	<u>book</u>	newspaper
7. train	<u>car</u>	bus
8. <u>suit</u>	pants	shirt
9. pitcher	cup	<u>glass</u>
10. <u>coat</u>	shirt	sweater

Set B

1.	bacon	<u>egg</u>	salt
2.	clock	<u>watch</u>	bracelet
3.	<u>salt</u>	sugar	pepper
4.	tulip	<u>rose</u>	vine
5.	glass	<u>cup</u>	mug
6.	suitcase	<u>box</u>	jar
7.	barn	<u>tent</u>	house
8.	clouds	sun	<u>sky</u>
9.	<u>milk</u>	water	coffee
10.	girl	man	<u>wife</u>

Level 3

Stimuli. Pictured nouns, unrelated series; grades 3 and 4 vocabulary; monosyllabic words

Set A		Set B	
1.	peach	1.	tea
2.	rug	2.	duck
3.	ball	3.	van
4.	nurse	4.	knife
5.	toast	5.	cat
6.	barn	6.	dish
7.	doll	7.	lamb
8.	sheet	8.	pen
9.	cake	9.	fence
10.	desk	10.	toy

Procedure. The following sets of three pictured nouns are placed in front of the patient. The clinician auditorily presents the underlined word and the patient points to the appropriate picture.

Set A

1.	<u>peach</u>	toy	lamb
2.	<u>rug</u>	tea	duck
3.	desk	<u>ball</u>	fence
4.	van	cat	<u>nurse</u>
5.	ball	<u>toast</u>	duck
6.	<u>barn</u>	knife	disk
7.	rug	peach	<u>doll</u>
8.	<u>sheet</u>	pen	van
9.	<u>cake</u>	ball	nurse
10.	fence	tea	<u>desk</u>

Set B

1.	cat	tea	lamb
2.	peach	duck	dish
3.	duck	doll	van
4.	knife	rug	barn
5.	cat	fence	pen
6.	dish	lamb	toy
7.	desk	lamb	toast
8.	rug	duck	pen
9.	knife	fence	nurse
10.	toy	cat	lamb

Additional Levels

Additional levels may be developed by altering the following parameters: word length, frequency of occurrence of words, semantic class, and grammatical class.

Area 5: Comprehension of Short Series

Beginning Levels

Level 1

Stimuli. Printed words, related series; grades 1 and 2 vocabulary; monosyllabic words: nouns and verbs

Procedure. The following sets of three printed words are placed in front of the patient. The clinician auditorily presents the words in a given row and the patient points to the appropriate series. If the patient is unable to read, pictured stimuli can be used.

Set A

1.	eat	drink	taste
	laugh	dance	sing
2.	stand	sit	fall
	break	tear	cut
3.	nose	arm	foot
	bag	case	box
4.	pay	sell	buy
	fight	beat	hurt
5.	train	car	ship
	queen	king	prince
6.	call	talk	say
	bring	pull	take
7.	paint	write	draw
	set	put	lay

8.	month	year	day
	south	north	west
9.	room	house	place
	ring	watch	gold
10.	seat	chair	bed
	star	sky	cloud

Set B

1.	snow	rain	ice
	shoe	size	foot
2.	come	go	stay
	see	watch	look
3.	learn	teach	show
	build	make	do
4.	catch	get	take
	know	think	feel
5.	food	cook	stove
	hat	head	hair
6.	hold	keep	have
	fly	drive	ride
7.	door	roof	floor
	road	town	stone
8.	wing	bird	tree
	lake	land	sky
9.	dream	bed	sleep
	day	night	time
10.	run	win	rush
	seek	find	lose

Level 2

Stimuli. Printed words, unrelated series; grades 1 and 2 vocabulary; monosyllabic words: nouns and verbs

Procedure. The following sets of three printed words are placed in front of the patient. The clinician auditorily presents the words in a given row and the patient points to the appropriate series.

Set A

1.	shoe	heart	farm
	view	job	car
2.	bear	leg	date
	game	height	milk
3.	spread	drink	take
	turn	wish	laugh

4. health	shape	month
voice	suit	chair
5. wait	hang	save
raise	press	sing
6. look	move	thank
stand	do	cut
7. shade	thing	news
shore	chief	gate
8. lay	sell	lose
spring	serve	want
9. march	save	guess
give	fall	paint
10. moon	girl	cup
top	blood	cent

Set B

1. page	bird	top
door	club	gold
2. blow	guide	catch
cost	stop	shape
3. heat	boy	piece
sign	clothes	word
4. man	street	week
knee	law	hall
5. press	drive	taste
beat	talk	add
6. kiss	gain	front
learn	join	lead
7. bill	fruit	pain
year	joy	sea
8. claim	live	hurt
work	miss	tell
9. bridge	art	food
meat	note	land
10. price	town	face
lie	war	yard

Level 3

Stimuli. Printed words, related series; grades 3 and 4 vocabulary; monosyllabic words: nouns and verbs

Procedure. The following series of three printed words are placed in front of the patient. The clinician auditorily presents the words in a given row and the patient points to the appropriate series.

Set A

1. pig   mouse   goat
   cake   bread   pie
2. truck   coach   van
   doll   block   ball
3. pinch   sting   bite
   leap   hop   jump
4. tea   juice   wine
   skirt   vest   shirt
5. choose pluck   seize
   praise   cheer   clap
6. knock   tap   hit
   preach bless   pray
7. cave   fort   hut
   bolt   screw   nail
8. dip   plunge   dive
   gaze   stare   glance
9. groan   sigh   gasp
   sew   mend   bind
10. plate   dish   pan
    cloth   silk   lace

Set B

1. throat   chin   cheek
   nest   straw   twig
2. clutch   seize   snatch
   grin   frown   wink
3. tread   crawl   trot
   mourn   grieve   weep
4. search   hunt   fetch
   slay   lash   whip
5. knife   fork   spoon
   mud   dirt   sand
6. chain   rope   string
   leaf   limb   trunk
7. snap   bend   split
   shriek   scream   yell
8. guest   priest   bride
   peach   plum   pear
9. vice   sin   crime
   soup   rice   beef
10. throw   pitch   toss
    pierce   dig   carve

Additional Levels

Additional levels may be developed by altering the following parameters: word length, frequency of occurrence of words, grammatical class, and semantic class. Word series will be easiest to process, followed by number series, phoneme series, and letter series.

Area 6: Comprehension of Short Meaningful Linguistic Units

Beginning Levels

Level 1

Stimuli. Action pictures; imperative sentences, three to five syllables; grades 1 and 2 vocabulary

Procedure. The clinician provides three pictured actions to the patient. An imperative sentence is auditorily presented by the clinician, with the patient requested to select the most appropriate picture.

Set A

1. Eat your food.
2. Drive the car.
3. Pay the bill.
4. Cut your meat.
5. Lift the box.
6. Sit on the chair.
7. Play the game.
8. Drink your milk.
9. Write your name.
10. Sell the house.

Set B

1. Press the dress.
2. Wash the clothes.
3. Go to the bank.
4. Watch the news.
5. Read the book
6. Spend your money.
7. Carry the baby.
8. Draw a picture.
9. Spread the butter.
10. Serve the dinner.

Level 2

Stimuli. Action pictures, imperative sentences, three to five syllables; grades 3 and 4 vocabulary

Procedure. The clinician provides three pictured actions to the patient. An imperative sentence is auditorily presented by the clincian, with the patient requested to select the most appropriate picture.

Set A

1. Polish the mirror.
2. Bake a cake.
3. Hit the nail.
4. Smell the pipe.
5. Melt the candle.
6. Lick the bowl.
7. Shut the trunk.

Set B

1. Rescue the driver.
2. Descend the stairs.
3. Carve the beef.
4. Repair the motor.
5. Upset the jar.
6. Climb over the fence.
7. Bite the candy.

8.	Chase the mouse.	8.	Fasten the rope.
9.	Fix the meal.	9.	Dig up the dirt.
10.	Collect the payment.	10.	Halt the traffic.

Level 3

Stimuli. Yes-no questions, three to five syllables; grades 1 and 2 vocabulary

Procedure. The following questions are presented auditorily and the patient is required to indicate "yes" or "no."

Set A

1. Do babies cry? (Y)
2. Can a dog learn? (Y)
3. Does a roof teach? (N)
4. Are people human? (Y)
5. Do flowers wonder? (N)
6. Can machines dance? (N)
7. Are birds rich? (N)
8. Can boards burn? (Y)
9. Can a child pray? (Y)
10. Is butter a fruit? (N)

Set B

1. Do plants grow? (Y)
2. Does a room travel? (N)
3. Do bridges wave? (N)
4. Can a leader lose? (Y)
5. Do lakes shop? (N)
6. Can a gun kill? (Y)
7. Do houses run? (N)
8. Are queens women? (Y)
9. Can doctors write? (Y)
10. Is sugar sweet? (Y)

Additional Levels

Additional levels may be developed by altering the following parameters: stimulus length, frequency of occurrence of words, sentence type, and topic familiarity.

Area 7: Comprehension of Sentences

Beginning Levels

Level 1

Stimuli. Pictured nouns; three to eight syllable sentences: simple active affirmative declarative with one independent clause; grades 1 and 2 vocabulary.

Procedure. Three pictured nouns are placed in front of the patient. The clinician auditorily presents a sentence with the last word omitted. The patient is requested to select the pictured word to complete the sentence.

Set A

1. The man builds _____. (houses)
2. The boy opened the _____. (door)
3. She talks on the _____. (telephone)
4. I prepared _____. (dinner)
5. He always burns the _____. (toast)
6. The cat broke the _____. (window)
7. We often walk to _____. (church)
8. I dried all the _____. (dishes)
9. My son spends too much _____. (money)
10. The man directed the _____. (cars)

Set B

1. My daughter reads strange _____. (books)
2. The dog killed the _____. (cat)
3. The child ran out of the _____. (house)
4. The boy caught the _____. (ball)
5. I always make my _____. (bed)
6. She pressed his _____. (pants)
7. Her husband washed his new _____. (car)
8. The mother kissed her _____. (baby)
9. The girl visits her _____. (grandmother)
10. The doctor sent a _____. (letter)

Level 2

Stimuli. Pictured nouns; 9 to 12 syllable sentences: simple active affirmative declarative with one independent clause; grades 1 and 2 vocabulary

Set A

1. The man paid for nine _____. (newspapers)
2. Our neighbor painted a pretty _____. (picture)
3. The president promised to build the _____. (bridge)
4. Today, the teacher traveled by _____. (train)
5. The building cost ten thousand _____. (dollars)
6. We kept the table in the _____. (kitchen)
7. My big brother became a _____. (soldier)
8. My daughter attempted to write a _____. (book)

9. It is important to water _____. (plants)
10. The gentleman forgot to mail the _____. (letter)

Set B

1. The company provided the _____. (milk)
2. Her good friend followed her to the _____. (church)
3. The daily newspaper is on the _____. (table)
4. During the winter, he painted his _____. (house)
5. For dinner he wants to eat fresh _____. (fish)
6. The beautiful flowers died in the _____. (rain)
7. Her husband is going to the _____. (farm)
8. His daughter discovered her shoes under the _____. (bed)
9. At the party, the man danced with his pretty _____. (wife)
10. His brother broke the fine _____. (watch)

Level 3

Stimuli. Pictured nouns; 9 to 12 syllable sentences: simple active affirmative declarative with an independent clause; grades 3 to 6 vocabulary

Set A

1. The policeman abandoned the _____. (painter)
2. The library had many books and _____. (magazines)
3. Joseph disliked professional _____. (football)
4. Everybody consumed the delicious _____. (candy)
5. The sailor assembled the _____. (compass)
6. Virginia ate a sandwich and a _____. (salad)
7. The clever fox confused the _____. (rabbit)
8. The hunter located the _____. (lion)
9. Elizabeth printed *Asia* on the _____. (map)
10. Robert blew out the birthday _____. (candles)

Set B

1. Dorothy fixed grandmother's broken _____. (plate)
2. Grandfather bought a canvas _____. (canoe)
3. Herbert hit a nail with a _____. (hammer)
4. The Canadian displayed Canada's _____. (flag)
5. We all went out for lunch to a _____. (restaurant)
6. Helen sewed the sleeve into the _____. (shirt)
7. The butcher distributed the _____. (beef)
8. Marvin carved the beef with a sharp _____. (knife)
9. I purchased a small bottle of _____. (perfume)
10. The dangerous animal growled at the _____. (mailman)

Additional Levels

Additional levels may be developed by altering the following parameters: stimulus length, sentence type, grammatical contrasts, and frequency of occurrence of words.

Area 8: Comprehension of Paragraphs

Beginning Levels

Level 1

Stimuli. Paragraphs: three sentences in length; 30 to 35 syllables; grades 1 to 4 vocabulary; yes-no questions

Procedure. The clinician reads aloud a paragraph, followed by both inferential and factual questions related to its content. The patient responds with "yes" or "no." To elicit 10 responses per set, two paragraphs are included in each set.

Set A

1. Mr. Black stopped at the store on his way home from work. He bought meat and fish. Mr. Black cooked the meat and saved the fish for the next day.

    a. Does Mr. Black have a job? (Y)
    b. Did Mr. Black go to the store on his way to work? (N)
    c. Did Mr. Black buy meat, fish, and milk? (N)
    d. Did Mr. Black cook the dinner? (Y)
    e. Did Mr. Black cook fish the next day? (Y)

2. My mother loves to work in the garden. Every spring she plants too many flowers. This year, we have no room for vegetables.

    a. Does my mother plant flowers in the fall? (N)
    b. Does my mother plant flowers every year? (Y)
    c. Are there many vegetables planted this year? (N)
    d. Does this story tell what types of flowers are planted? (N)
    e. Does this story tell how to grow a good garden? (N)

Set B

1. Each Christmas, I like to give a party. All of my friends are invited. There is always lots of food, soft music, and good conversation.

    a. Do I visit with friends at Christmas? (Y)
    b. Do I invite all of the people from the office to my party? (N)
    c. Do I usually run out of food at the party? (N)

    d.   Do the neighbors object to the music? (N)
    e.   Do the parties appear to be pleasant? (Y)

2. My daughter is old enough to learn to drive. I want her to take
    lessons but my husband is going to teach her. I hope they use his
    car.
    a.   Am I a single woman? (N)
    b.   Is my daughter five years old? (N)
    c.   Do I want to teach my daughter how to drive? (N)
    d.   Is my husband a driving teacher? (N)
    e.   Do I have a car? (Y)

Level 2

Stimuli. Paragraphs: four sentences in length; 60 to 70 syllables;
grades 1 to 4 vocabulary; yes-no questions

Procedure. The clinician reads aloud a paragraph, followed by both
inferential and factual questions related to its content. The patient responds with "yes" or "no." Only one paragraph is included in each set to
elicit 10 responses, at this level.

Set A

Whenever I walk in the rain without a coat, I get a bad head cold. I
hate to wait in line at the doctor's office. Instead, I stay home from work
and hardly get out of bed. With plenty of rest, lots of hot tea, and good
books, I feel better, just over night.

1.   Do I ever get colds from the rain? (Y)
2.   Do I work in a doctor's office? (N)
3.   Do I ask the doctor to visit me at home? (N)
4.   Do I ever miss work? (Y)
5.   Do I refuse to stay in bed when I'm sick? (N)
6.   Do hot drinks make me feel better? (Y)
7.   Do I write letters when I'm sick? (N)
8.   Does it take a long time for me to get better? (N)
9.   Do I go to my mother's when I'm sick? (N)
10. Do I take good care of myself when I'm sick? (Y)

Set B

In the late summer, our family likes to go to the lake. We usually rent a
cabin near the water. My husband enjoys getting up early, going for a boat
ride and then preparing breakfast. It's about the only time of year our
children stay in bed until nine o'clock.

1.   Does our whole family go on our trip? (Y)
2.   Does our family like to take our trip in June? (N)
3.   Do we own a cabin? (N)

4. Does my husband like the water? (Y)
5. Does my husband like to sleep late? (N)
6. Do our children usually get up early? (Y)
7. Do I do all the cooking on our trip? (N)
8. Does my husband run before breakfast? (N)
9. Does the story say that my husband is a good cook? (N)
10. Does this story say that our children stay up late at night? (N)

Level 3

Stimuli. Paragraphs: three sentences in length; 30 to 35 syllables; grades 5 and 6 vocabulary; yes-no questions

Procedure. The clinician reads aloud a paragraph, followed by both inferential and factual questions related to its content. The patient responds with "yes" or "no." To elicit 10 responses per set, two paragraphs are included in each set.

Set A

1. The tourist napped on the beach, with his camera. The clumsy thief inspected his baggage. Fortunately, a wasp distracted the amateur.
    a. Does this story take place near the water? (Y)
    b. Was the tourist sleepy? (Y)
    c. Was the thief a professional? (N)
    d. Did the tourist scare the thief? (N)
    e. Did the thief take the camera? (N)
2. We had all the ingredients for a hearty picnic. Thoughtfully, we devised a menu. Then we sped to the waterfall on bicycles.
    a. Did we go to the beach? (N)
    b. Did we travel on foot? (N)
    c. Did we take food with us? (Y)
    d. Did we have a lot of food? (Y)
    e. Did we hurry to our destination? (Y)

Set B

1. For leisure, the bachelor makes pastry. He modifies recipes to perfection. A tray of his baking dazzles even his housekeeper.
    a. Is this story about a professional baker? (N)
    b. Does the bachelor dislike baking? (N)
    c. Does the bachelor bake without a recipe? (N)
    d. Does someone help the bachelor look after his house? (Y)
    e. Does the housekeeper like the bachelor's pastry? (Y)
2. As a pastime, I study the violin. I sometimes falter on Beethoven's melodies. I hope to excel by Thanksgiving.

a. Do I play the violin? (Y)
b. Do I study the violin for leisure? (Y)
c. Do I have difficulty with Beethoven's music? (Y)
d. Does the story say that I practice for 20 minutes a day? (N)
e. Is this a story about a Thanksgiving celebration? (N)

Additional Levels

Additional levels may be developed by altering the following parameters: length of sentences, syntactic complexity of sentences, frequency of occurrence of words, degree of topic familiarity, degree of patient interest in topic, amount of content (facts), and cohesion among sentence units.

Area 9: Comprehension of Narratives and Discourse

Beginning Levels

Level 1

Stimuli. Newspaper articles; 60 to 80 syllables in length; high degree of cohesion among sentence units; limited number of facts; yes-no questions

Procedure. The article is read aloud by the clinician, followed by both inferential and factual questions related to its content. The patient responds with "yes" or "no."

Set A

MANAMA, Bahrain (Reuter)—One person was killed and three were injured when charges of dynamite planted in two garbage cans exploded last night in a street in the Saudi Arabia city of Riyadh, the Saudi news agency SPA reported. The agency did not say who was responsible for the explosion.

1. Were more than one person injured in this story? (Y)
2. Were there any fatalities in the explosion? (Y)
3. Were any of the injuries related to gunfire? (N)
4. Was dynamite found behind a garbage can? (N)
5. Did the dynamite explode during the afternoon? (N)
6. Did this story take place in Saudi Arabia? (Y)
7. Was this story reported by a Saudi news agency? (Y)
8. Is SPA the name of a terrorist group? (N)
9. Is Riyadh a city in Saudi Arabia? (Y)
10. Were people arrested in connection with the explosion? (N)

Set B

DETROIT (AP)—Several groups have cancelled reservations at a suburban hotel where 30 people are believed to have contracted Legionnaires' disease, even though health authorities say there is little chance of another outbreak of the respiratory illness.

1. Is this a story about tuberculosis? (N)
2. Is the hotel located in downtown Detroit? (N)
3. Is the hotel's business affected by the outbreak of the disease? (Y)
4. Have more than a dozen people been stricken with the disease? (Y)
5. Have health officials been notified? (Y)
6. Has the hotel been quarantined? (N)
7. Are health officials concerned about the possibility of a widespread epidemic? (N)
8. Have health officials suggested a boycott of the hotel? (N)
9. Does this article say that Legionnaires' disease is not contagious? (N)
10. Is Legionnaires' disease a respiratory illness? (Y)

Level 2

Stimuli. Weather forecasts; 80 to 120 syllables in length; high degree of cohesion among sentence units; several facts; multiple choice questions

Procedure. The forecast is read aloud by the clinician, followed by multiple choice questions related to its content. The questions may be presented auditorily or in written form, depending on the skills of the patient. The patient either orally provides a response or points to a written choice. In order to elicit 10 responses at this level, two forecasts are included.

Set A

FORECAST
Cloudy skies with the chance of showers early today are expected to be replaced by mostly sunny skies after noon when a weak disturbance moves across Southwestern Ontario. A high of 55 and a low of 17 are forecast. Northwest winds are expected at 18 to 25 miles per hour. There's a 20 percent chance of precipitation.

1. Skies will be
   a. cloudy
   b. variable throughout the day
2. Chance of rain is
   a. greater than 50 percent
   b. less than 50 percent
3. Winds will be
   a. from the northwest
   b. from the southeast

4. The high temperature will be
   a. in the fifties
   b. in the forties
5. The low temperature will be
   a. below freezing
   b. above freezing

FORECAST

A low pressure system moving in from Michigan is causing showers, rain and drizzle at different times throughout the day along with northwest winds of 9 to 15 miles per hour. The probability of precipitation is listed at 80 percent, and the high is expected to reach 58. Tonight's low is forecast at 50. Normal highs and lows for this date are 66 and 45.

1. It will rain
   a. only in the morning
   b. throughout the day
2. Chance of rain is
   a. greater than 50 percent
   b. less than 50 percent
3. A low pressure area is coming from
   a. New York
   b. Michigan
4. The high temperature will be
   a. in the fifties
   b. in the seventies
5. The low temperature will be
   a. below freezing
   b. above freezing

Set B

FORECAST

Cloudy skies with afternoon showers are expected today as a low pressure system moves east across the upper Great Lakes and Georgian Bay areas. A high of 68 and a low of 48 are forecast with light to moderate southwest winds at 13 to 19 miles per hour. The chance of rain is rated at 30 percent.

1. Skies will be
   a. clear
   b. cloudy
2. Chance of rain is
   a. greater than 50 percent
   b. less than 50 percent

3. Winds will be
   a. high
   b. light to moderate
4. The high temperature will be
   a. in the seventies
   b. in the sixties
5. The low temperature will be
   a. in the forties
   b. in the twenties

   FORECAST
   A cool front moving into Southwestern Ontario is expected to replace this morning's showers and mild weather with clearing skies and lower temperatures. A high of 70 and a low of 50 are forecast, with southwest winds at 20 to 28 miles per hour this morning diminishing and shifting to northwesterly breezes at 10 to 15 miles per hour by late this afternoon. The probability of precipitation is rated at 70 percent.

1. Skies will be
   a. clear
   b. variable throughout the day
2. Chance of rain is
   a. greater than 50 percent
   b. less than 50 percent
3. Winds will be
   a. increasing over the day
   b. diminishing over the day
4. The high temperature will be
   a. in the sixties
   b. in the seventies
5. The low temperature will be
   a. below freezing
   b. above freezing

   Level 3

   Stimuli. Horoscope; 30 to 40 syllables in length; low degree of cohesion among sentence units; several facts, yes-no questions

   Procedure. The horoscope is read aloud by the clinician, followed by both inferential and factual questions related to its content. The patient responds with "yes" or "no." In order to elicit 10 responses at this level, two horoscopes have been included in each set.

Set A

   Leo (July 23–Aug. 22): Accent on authority, achievement, responsibility, money, intensified love relationship. Desires are fulfilled, advancement occurs in career.

1. Does this horoscope focus on both career and personal life? (Y)
2. Does this horoscope say you will lose a large amount of money? (N)
3. Will your career be positively affected? (Y)
4. Will your love life be enhanced? (Y)
5. Does the horoscope predict more travel? (N)

Sagittarius (Nov. 22–Dec. 21): Go slow, check trends, keep resolulutions concerning physical appearance, diet. Demands are made on your time as social activities increase.

1. Does this horoscope advise caution? (Y)
2. Does this horoscope say that you will stray from your diet? (N)
3. Will your social life become busier? (Y)
4. Will you have more free time? (N)
5. Will more demands be made on you because of your work? (N)

Set B

Piscces (Feb. 19-March 20): Check home for safety hazards—remove them. Emphasis on security, conclusion of transaction, reunion with long-standing associate.

1. Will greater emphasis be placed on your friendships? (N)
2. Does the horoscope warn of possible danger? (Y)
3. Is a reunion with a family member suggested? (N)
4. Will a transaction be completed? (Y)
5. Will you be meeting with someone that you have known for a long time? (Y)

Virgo (Aug. 23–Sept. 22): Reach beyond current expectations—you are going to be surprised by enthusiastic reception. Past favors are repaid, more people are drawn to you.

1. Does this horoscope suggest that you be daring? (Y)
2. Will you receive an enthusiastic response from others? (Y)
3. Does the horoscope say that you will be disappointed by your friends? (N)
4. Will you be repaying past favors? (N)
5. Will your popularity increase? (Y)

Additional Levels

Additional levels may be developed to include television and radio segments, followed by a test of the patient's comprehension. The following parameters may be varied: stimulus length, degree of topic familiarity, degree of patient interest in topic, amount of content (facts), and cohesion among sentence units.

APPENDIX 3-1

REFERENCES FOR PICTURE MATERIALS

Blockolsky, V. D., Frazer, J. M., Kurn, B. A., and Metz, F. E. (1977). *Peel and put pictures.* Communication Skill Builders (Division of Moyer Vico, Weston, Ont.).

Dunn, L. M., and Smith, J. O. (1966). *Peabody language development kits: Level 2.* American Guidance Service (Division of Psychan Ltd., Willowdale, Ont.).

Dunn, L. M., and Smith, J. O. (1967). *Peabody language development kits: Level 3.* American Guidance Service (Division of Psychan Ltd., Willowdale, Ont.).

Familiar sounds. (1972). Developmental Learning Materials (Division of PMB Industries, Scarborough, Ont.).

Hain, R., and Lainer, H. (1977). *Language rehabilitation program: Level 1.* Teaching Resources Corp. (Division of Ginn & Company, Scarborough, Ont.).

Hain, R., and Lainer, H. (1980). *Language rehabilitation program: Level 2.* Teaching Resources Corp. (Division of Ginn & Company, Scarborough, Ont.).

Medlin, W. L. (1975). *Word making cards.* Salt Lake City, UT: Word Making Productions.

Taylor, M. L., and Marks, M. M. (1959). *Aphasia rehabilitation and therapy kit.* Scarborough, Ont.: McGraw-Hill Ryerson.

Chapter 4

Treatment for Visual Processing

As with auditory comprehension deficits, all aphasic patients demonstrate difficulties with reading comprehension. The severity of the deficit varies, but in general the severity of the reading disorder parallels that for auditory comprehension (Duffy and Ulrich, 1976; Van Demark, Lemmer, and Drake, 1982) and is highly correlated with the overall severity of the language disorder in chronic aphasic patients (Van Demark et al., 1982; Webb and Love, 1983). In contrast to auditory comprehension, which all persons need in order to function in an auditory world, reading comprehension skills may be less vital to some patients. Therefore, the clinician and patient will need to decide to what extent treatment will include visual processing deficits. Typically, our clinical experience has been that treatment will include some work with this modality to permit aphasic patients to exercise functional reading if that is their maximal potential or desire. Of less importance now, but certainly relevant in past decades, is the illiterate aphasic patient for whom reading treatment is inappropriate. A case history should provide the clinician with information about literacy.

Various types of visual processing and reading deficits occur in patients who have suffered cerebral lesions. Reading disturbance is not a unitary disorder and this must be accounted for in treatment. Many of these deficits have carried the term alexia, modified by one or more adjectives (e.g., pure alexia, agnosic alexia, aphasic alexia). Some of these deficits occur in aphasic patients; others do not and these are specified as strictly not being accompanied by significant aphasia.

Perhaps it is most appropriate to begin with definitions. *Alexia* is a term generally used to refer to an inability to comprehend written material following cerebral insult. Therefore, it refers to acquired reading disorders and not to developmental dyslexia, which should be ruled out prior to initiating treatment with the adult aphasic patient. This definition has been adopted by many prominent aphasiologists, such as Geschwind, Benson (Benson and Geschwind, 1969; Benson, 1979), and Damasia (1977).
Since all aphasic patients have reading comprehension deficits to a greater or lesser degree (Webb and Love, 1983), we might say that all aphasic patients are alexic. The term alexia, however, is applied to aphasic patients only when the reading disturbance coincides with a particular pattern. Therefore, all aphasic patients have reading deficits; some reading deficits in aphasic patients have been labeled alexic (e.g., frontal alexia in Broca's aphasic patients), some alexias occur in isolation (e.g, alexia without agraphia), and some are accompanied by aphasia. Figure 4–1 shows the relationship between aphasia and alexia. This chapter will focus primarily on those reading deficits found in aphasic patients, with reference to alexia when appropriate.

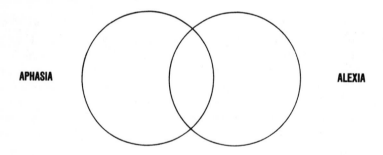

Figure 4–1.   This figure indicates the overlapping nature of aphasic disorders and alexic disorders.

Although not germane to the content of this chapter but to complete the definition of alexia, the term has been used and is currently used today to refer to disturbances of oral reading. As such, the terms pure alexia, phonemic alexia, surface dyslexia, and deep dyslexia are frequently seen in the literature (Coltheart, 1982; Coltheart, Patterson, and Marshall, 1980; Marshall and Newcombe, 1973; Saffran and Marin, 1977).

Oral reading deficits will be covered in a subsequent chapter. Suffice it here to alert the clinician to the terminological morass and to delineate the boundaries of the present discussion.

Visual processing, as a language modality, involves the processing of information presented visually, which can include both pictorial material and written language. The treatment guidelines here have followed the same principle as for auditory processing, that of dividing deficits into two major categories, those that pertain to visual perceptual deficits and those that involve reading comprehension deficits. Although perceptual deficits may not be a primary factor contributing to reading problems, when present, they can negatively influence reading test performance. Webb and Love (1983) reported that the presence of visual field deficits was associated with significantly more errors on a reading test. Some perceptual training may be necessary before a patient with severe reading deficits can approach comprehension tasks.

TYPES OF VISUAL PROCESSING DEFICITS

Visual Processing Deficits in Aphasia

The reading process requires perceptual processing prior to achieving comprehension of visual material. Therefore, if visual perceptual processing is disturbed such that an aphasic patient cannot discriminate material or recognize its class membership, comprehension of the visual material will not be possible. Although aphasic patients do have difficulty with both recognition and comprehension tasks, the latter tasks evoke more errors (Schuell et al., 1964; Webb and Love, 1983).

Visual Perceptual Deficits

On aphasia test batteries, aphasic patients, particularly those with more severe language deficits, make errors on tasks involving visual recognition. They may fail to discriminate accurately and fail to match objects, drawings, forms, colors, letters, words, and so on (Schuell, 1964; Varney, 1981). They may have difficulty recognizing the correspondence between different letters or words written in different scripts (Goodglass and Kaplan, 1983; Kaplan and Goodglass, 1981; Varney, 1981) or in recognizing nonverbal visual patterns, such as trademarks (Gardner, 1974a; Wapner and Gardner, 1981). Schuell and co-workers (1964) reported spatial disorientation interfering with reading in the "aphasic with scattered findings" group, although it should be noted that these patients had bilateral lesions.

Aphasic patients also may have difficulty recognizing visual symbols in a variety of categories, such as numbers, colors, objects, punctuation marks, faces, and so on (Gardner, 1974a). When shown members of these categories visually, aphasic groups, and particularly the posterior ones, made more errors in recognizing the correct name presented by the examiner. Even when aphasic individuals did not have to associate the name with the visual symbol, they showed some recognition difficulties (Wapner and Gardner, 1981).

Because visual acuity and visual field deficits do influence visual performance (Webb and Love, 1983), they should be accounted for during any visual testing. Visual attention, scanning, and tracking problems are frequent in patients with right hemisphere lesions but should also be ruled out as potential underlying problems during visual perceptual and reading tasks with left hemisphere–damaged aphasic patients. Should they occur, they should be remedied with appropriate treatment.

Visual Comprehension Problems

In most aphasic patients visual comprehension problems will involve comprehension of the written word. However, for some patients with extremely severe auditory comprehension problems, an alternate or augmentative gestural communication system may be used, such as Amer-Ind (Skelly, 1979). Gestures vary in their degree of symbolism, with some being iconic and others being symbolic. Gestures can also be sequenced to create a more complex message. Some systems, such as American Sign Language (ASL), form a language; others, such as Amer-Ind, are sign systems only.

Reading comprehension problems, present in aphasic patients, vary in both type and severity (Albert, Goodglass, Helm, Rubens, and Alexander, 1981). Short and easy material is generally comprehended with fewer errors than long and complicated material. Less frequently occurring words in addition to abstract, nonoperative, non-noun words are comprehended less accurately than common, concrete, operative nouns (Schuell et al., 1964; Gardner and Zurif, 1976; Albert et al., 1981). Therefore, frequency, concreteness, and part of speech influence a patient's performance on single-word tasks.

Length of material also affects comprehension, whether at a sentence or a paragraph level. Clinically, it is well known that it is the exceptional aphasic patient who can return to reading short stories or novels let alone more technical material. As individual paragraphs increase in length, aphasic patients make more comprehension errors (Schuell et al., 1964), although length and redundancy have reportedly been beneficial to some Wernicke's aphasic patients (Albert et al., 1981).

Complexity of written material can be increased by varying the syntactic structure. Broca's aphasic patients seem particularly vulnerable to material increased in difficulty via this method (Albert et al., 1981; Caramazza et al., 1981a; Kaplan and Goodglass, 1981), although other aphasic patients make more errors on more complex material when general complexity measures, such as grade level equivalents, are used (Van Demark et al., 1982).

Posterior Alexia (Occipital Alexia, Alexia without Agraphia)

Loss of or impaired ability to read with preserved spontaneous writing and writing to dictation are the defining symptoms of alexia without agraphia (Ajax, Schenkenberg, and Kosteljanetz, 1977; Benson, 1979; Benson, Brown, and Tomlinson, 1971; Benson and Geschwind, 1969; Damasio, 1977; Stachowiak and Pöeck, 1976; Vincent, Sadowsky, Saunders, and Reeves, 1977). The syndrome is most often associated with vascular causes, particularly thrombosis of the posterior cerebral artery resulting in a lesion to the left visual cortex and the splenium of the corpus callosum. Rare are those cases of alexia without agraphia due to tumor (Cohen, Salanga, Hully, Steinberg, and Hardy, 1976) or trauma (Staller, Buchanan, Singer, Lappin, and Webb, 1978). Frequently, reported symptoms accompanying the syndrome are right homonymous hemianopsia, a color naming deficit, inability to read musical notes and numbers, and a calculation disorder, although these are not invariably present (Ajax, 1967; Cumming, Hurwitz, and Perl, 1970). Some cases have also noted defective object naming and defective typographical orientation. These patients are not aphasic but have difficulty comprehending written material. Most typically, subjects are described as having difficulty recognizing words although their letter recognition is better. Therefore, they attempt to comprehend a word using an analytical approach, spelling it letter by letter (Ajax, 1967; Stachowiak and Pöeck, 1976; Staller et al., 1978). Of course, the longer the word, the more time this takes, and reading longer and complex material is impossible. Benson and Geschwind refer to this type as the verbal subtype of alexia with agraphia and it is analogous to Hécaen and Kremin's (1976) verbal alexia. In a small number of cases, patients with this syndrome reportedly recognized some words but had relatively more difficulty with letter recognition (Benson and Geschwind, 1969; Hécaen and Kremin, 1976; Lecours, L'hermitte, and Bryans, 1983). This symptom is referred to as the literal subtype by Benson and Geschwind (1969) and as literal alexia by Hécaen and Kremin (1976). In later versions of Benson's work (1979) this subtype was deleted. Although Benson and Geschwind pointed out that patients with alexia without agraphia rarely have only one subtype but rather present both symptoms with one predominating, Benson's later work (1979) indicates that verbal alexia is predominant.

The writing of these patients, both spontaneously and to dictation, although not perfect, is remarkably better than their reading. Although they can copy words, ruling out visual perceptual deficits, they do so very slowly and laboriously. Another distinguishing feature of these patients is their ability to read using input from other modalities. For example, they can understand words traced on their palms and can read a word by tracing it (Cumming et al., 1970) using tactile information. Acoustic cues and pictures (visual cues) (Stachowiak and Pöeck, 1976) are also helpful.

Prognosis for the recovery of the reading disorder in these patients has been mixed. Ajax (1967) reported little change in his two patients. Cueing via other modalities (sometimes also referred to as deblocking techniques) have been helpful to other patients (Stachowiak and Pöeck, 1976; Staller et al., 1978).

Central Alexia (Parietal-Temporal Alexia, Alexia with Agraphia)

This syndrome is characterized by the loss of the ability both to read and to write, usually as a result of a lesion to the parietal-temporal area or the dominant angular gyrus. Although the cause is frequently vascular (posterior branch of the middle cerebral artery), it may also be traumatic or neoplastic. The reading disturbance is severe, involves both literal and verbal alexias, may include numbers, musical notes, and frequently a severe calculation deficit. Input from other modalities does not help the reading, as was the case for alexia without agraphia. The writing disturbance is severe and, with the reading deficit, renders the patients illiterate. These patients cannot recognize spelled words nor can they spell words orally. (A case that was an exception to this has been reported by Rothi and Heilman [1981].) They have difficulty copying and may demonstrate an associated Gerstmann syndrome.

This syndrome can occur in isolation but may be associated with aphasia, usually Wernicke's aphasia.

Frontal Alexia (Literal Alexia)

This variety of alexia, described by Benson (1977, 1979), presents itself as a reading disturbance in which the recognition of letters is extremely impaired although the patient can read some words, primarily substantive ones. The severity of the alexia, predominantly of the literal variety, increases with less frequently occurring letters, structurally more complex ones, phonetically similar letters, and visually similar letters (Hécaen and Kremin, 1976; Lecours et al., 1983). Patients may be able to read some words using a global approach and some short sentences. In the latter case, they appear to rely on the substantive words to derive meaning, rather than on syntactic processing (Benson, 1979; Caramazza, Berndt, and Hart, 1981b). These patients may recognize some words spelled aloud although they have limited success and perform poorly on spelling words aloud.

A severe writing disturbance is almost always present, characterized by poorly formed letters and incorrect spelling. Copying is possible, but achieved with much greater difficulty than the two previously described alexias.

This syndrome is usually accompanied by Broca's aphasia. Frequent accompanying symptoms are right hemiparesis and a visual field defect. As with Broca's aphasia the cause is vascular in the majority of cases, in the form of a lesion to the posterior portion of the inferior frontal gyrus with extensions to the underlying subcortical tissues of the anterior insula.

Visual Agnosia

Visual agnosia, a rare syndrome, occurs when a patient is unable to recognize material presented visually (Benson and Geschwind, 1969; Eisenson, 1984) that is recognizable when presented via other modalities. The patient generally uses the name in spoken language but cannot name it on visual confrontation. Failure to recognize occurs across several categories of material, both verbal (printed and written words, letters, and so on) and nonverbal (forms, objects, and so forth). Two types of visual agnosia, apperceptive and associative, have been described. The former corresponds to bilateral lesions to the striate cortex and surrounding visual association areas, often due to vascular insufficiency. These patients fail to recognize and name visually presented material. Nor can they copy visual objects, letters, and so on because of the bilateral visual cortex destruction. Of course, these patients cannot copy written language and they cannot read. Since writing is maintained, visual agnosic patients demonstrate alexia without agraphia. However, it should be noted that visual agnosia should not be construed as the general cause of the former syndrome. Reported associated findings to visual agnosia have been constructional apraxia, right homonymous hemianopsia, prosopagnosia, amnesia, and naming difficulties (Benson and Greenberg, 1969). Benson (1979) hypothesized that visual agnosia is more common than can be demonstrated because it may be masked by aphasia, particularly Wernicke's aphasia.

GENERAL GUIDELINES FOR VISUAL PROCESSING TREATMENT

The two major categories within the visual processing modality have been subdivided into mutually exclusive areas for the reasons outlined in the previous chapter. Which areas are selected for treatment is determined by the clinician, often in a joint decision with the patient, based on the patient's test performance and interests. It is also important to consider the patient's educational level as several authors have reported substantial influences of education on reading performance (Porch, 1971; Schuell, Jenkins, and Landis, 1961; Webb and Love, 1983). Since reading disturbance is not a single entity in aphasia, it is necessary to delineate the problem for each individual and to direct treatment to it.

The following treatment guidelines for visual processing deficits will help clinicians establish treatment hierarchies to enable a patient to progress from an initial level to a maximal potential reading level. The hierarchies have been based on information in the literature about acquired reading deficits as a result of cerebral insult. Detailed attention to the study of reading and to its treatment are relatively recent in the research literature. Therefore, future research promises to add to the data base presented here.

Area 1: Matching Nonverbal Material

1. Identical Materials

Stimuli. Matching nonverbal materials does not deal with language tasks per se. However, some severely impaired aphasic patients demonstrate difficulty with even the simplest language tasks (Helm and Benson, 1978; Porch, 1981). For these patients it is important to start treatment with tasks that they can perform. In the case of visual processing, matching tasks are the easiest.

Specific parameters of matching tasks have not been systematically investigated in aphasia, probably due, at least in part, to the ability of most patients to accomplish these tasks without error. Information from other modalities would suggest that concreteness, familiarity, and operativity are important parameters to consider, with the easiest tasks involving highly familiar, concrete, operative materials.

In general, objects will be easier to match than pictures, as evidenced by the rank ordering of these tasks on the PICA (Porch, 1981). The difficulty of the matching tasks designed will depend on the aforementioned parameters. In addition, the complexity of pictures and the degree of stylization may affect matching performance, with photographic representations being easier than stylized representations.

Whether two dimensional geometric shapes are more difficult than pictures is unknown. Baseline testing with the individual aphasic patient can best determine where to place these materials in a hierarchy of tasks. The following is suggested:

Easy	Objects
↓	Pictures
Difficult	Geometric forms

Size of the materials should be adequate such that errors in matching are not made on the basis of visual acuity problems.

Description. The activities within this area are designed to have the aphasic patient focus on the visual parameters of materials—to discriminate whether they are alike or different. Categorization or understanding of the materials is not required for these tasks, as the emphasis is on visual discrimination skills. The purpose of these tasks is to have the aphasic patient attend to and process visual material.

Example. The aphasic patient matches identical objects used in a table setting (knife, fork, spoon, plate, cup, and so on).

2. Nonidentical Materials

Stimuli. In these matching tasks, an added dimension is class recognition, because the items to be matched are no longer identical. Therefore, the aphasic patient must recognize that two differently shaped cups match because they belong to the same category.

Easy	Objects
↓	Pictures
Difficult	Geometric forms

Variables to Control
Number of response choices
Class membership
Visual similarity
Number of dimensions

These tasks can be increased in difficulty by altering the response array available to the patient. A larger number of choices may make the task more difficult. Having all choices belong to similar semantic classes as well as the number of dimensions of similarity or contrast can increase task difficulty. The more visually similar are the choices the greater attention will be required for the aphasic individual to select the appropriate match.

Description. These tasks are designed to have the aphasic patient attend to the visual modality, to make discriminations, and to demonstrate recognition of a common category membership.

Example. The aphasic patient matches a series of pictures in which the pictures of each pair are visually different but belong to the same category. Given ten cards with domestic animals, the patient matches the animals in the same category (e.g., collie—spaniel: dog; Siamese—calico: cat; and so on).

Area 2: Matching Verbal Material

1. Single Items

Stimuli. Numbers, letters, and words compose the verbal materials included in this area. These are the individual elements, along with punctuation, that make up the written language code. At this time, evidence does not exist of a clear hierarchy of difficulty among the three categories when other variables are controlled, such as length and visual similarity. For some aphasic patients (with pure alexia) longer items may precipitate more errors and, among words, words that are more similar visually may precipitate more errors than visually dissimilar items on match-to-sample tasks (Filby, Edwards, and Seacat, 1963).

> Numbers
> Letters
> Words
>
> **Variables to Control**
> Length
> Visual similarity
> Size of stimuli

Description. The activities in this area are designed to promote visual attention to and discrimination of the categories that compose the written language code. In this area it it not necessary for the aphasic individual to comprehend the items but only to recognize the visual similarities and differences.

Example. The aphasic patient performs a match-to-sample task. Shown a written word (e.g., hat), the patient matches it with its identical counterpart, given a choice of two written words (e.g., hat, ring).

2. Series of Items

Stimuli. Stimuli are the same categories as for single items. In this area the aphasic patient processes items in a series, rather than processing single items. The categories, as previously, are not hierarchically arranged:

> Number series
> Letter series
> Word series

Description. The serial items require the aphasic patient to process more material. In that respect, they are similar to reading comprehension tasks and serve as a precursor to them. With the increased amount of material, memory and attention span are more heavily taxed than in tasks with single items.

Example. The aphasic patient is shown a series of three numbers for 5 seconds. The number series is removed and the patient selects the matching number series from a choice of three. An easier version of this task leaves the series in view during the selection process.

Area 3: Visual Correspondence-Recognition

1. Association of Visual Materials

Stimuli. The stimuli in this area consist of various combinations of the classes that compose the written language code—letters, words, and numbers. With recognition tasks, the aphasic patient must recognize the correspondence of items in different visual forms and recognize their class membership. Often the tasks in this area require the matching of printed words with pictures or objects, printed number words with their ciphers, and letters in different forms.

Some categories of visual forms are easier than others for aphasic patients. The hierarchy below, listed from easy to difficult, is that found by Wapner and Gardner (1981) for a task in which subjects had to select the correct symbol from an array of four. Williams and Owens's (1977) finding that recall of pictures was easier than recall of printed words in aphasic patients corroborates Wapner and Gardner's data.

	Category	Example
Easy	Trademarks I	Recognition of correct symbol
	Pictured objects	(American eagle, NBC peacock)
	Number related symbols	$(+, -, \$)$
	Word-picture	(One word—four pictures)
	Trademarks II	
	Pictorial logo	**Camel** on package of cigarettes
	Abbreviation	**L** and **M** on package of cigarettes
	Whole name	**Winston** on package of cigarettes
Difficult	Traffic signs	

Broca's aphasic patients performed better than Wernicke's aphasic subjects although the hierarchies of difficulty for both groups were similar.

Recognition of categories of numbers, letters, colors, and animals was performed well by most aphasic patients (Gardner, 1974a), and no hierarchy of difficulty was provided. Gardner did mention that global aphasic individuals performed the worst, and posterior aphasic subjects performed significantly worse than an anterior lesion group. It should be noted that recognition was tested such that the aphasic patient selected from a group of three choices spoken by the examiner. Therefore, the task was not limited to the visual modality.

Letter strings that form English words and strings that do not form words can be used in lexical decision tasks to determine if the aphasic patient can recognize words in the language. Several patterns of responding were found but the following hierarchy held (Friedman, 1981).

	Category	Example
Easy	Letter strings	Orthographically irregular, nonpronounceable (bdxc)
	Real words	Orthographically regular, pronounceable (help)
	Pseudowords	Orthographically regular, prounounceable (felp)
Difficult		

Difficulty can vary with any category presented for visual recognition. For example, certain letters and letter forms are easier than others. Lecours and co-workers (1983) found that literal alexic patients (often with Broca's aphasia) had more difficulty recognizing complex letters than simple ones, and several factors influenced their recognition performance.

Easy	Structural Complexity	Visual Similarity	Phonetic Similarity
↓	O, I, L	M, E	p, s
Difficult	G, H, F	M, N	p, b

Variables to Control
Size of letter
Orientation of letter
Duration of exposure
Background against which letters are exposed

Description. The activites in this area are desgined to aid the aphasic patient in the symbolic recognition of visual material, pictorial symbols, or orthographic symbols. These tasks extend beyond visual discrimination to identification and therefore require the patient to recognize the item presented in another form as the same symbol. Therefore, the patient must recognize the correspondence between different visual forms and be able to assign class membership. That is, the patient must appreciate the identity of individual letters and their equivalences across different scripts.

Although no group significant differences were found for printed versus script single words identification, Williams (1984) reported marked differences for individual patients. Therefore, this is important to check prior to treatment. Another type of stimulus category is numbers, and whether aphasic patients can identify word-cipher correspondences is another kind of task to include.

Example. The aphasic patient matches a given picture (hat) with the appropriate picture from an array of four. The choices are the correct response (different type of hat), a semantically associated response (coat), an acoustically similar response (bat), and a visually similar response (an upside-down cup on a saucer).

2. Association of Materials within a Superordinate Category

Stimuli. The stimuli in this area are nonverbal visual stimuli that may be related to one another in a variety of ways. The stimuli may be related members of a particular semantic category or they may be in a subordinate-superordinate relationship. Semantic categories like those discussed for auditory comprehension can be used, and 54 different categories and their most frequent members can be found in Battig and Montague (1969).

Description. These tasks are designed to prompt association of visual nonverbal materials in particular relationships. They are set up to require the aphasic patient to abstract a relationship between two or more objects or pictures.

Example. A pair of pictures, a baseball and a baseball mitt, as well as a picture of a basketball, are shown. From another array of three pictures the aphasic patient selects the once that demonstrates the analogous relationship to that between the baseball and mitt, that is, a basketball hoop.

Area 4: Reception of Gestured Messages

Usually aphasic patients depend on auditory comprehension, reading skills, or both to decode messages. These are not the only modalities through which messages may be received. Pictures are another form of stimulus that can convey messages, as are gestures. Both involve visual processing skills and this area will focus on the reception of gestured messages.

At this point it is important to note that gesture or nonverbal behavior can occur in several forms, and researchers have studied these various forms. Gesture may refer to motor behavior that accompanies speech, such as facial expression (mimicry), or to body or hand movements (gesticulation). Gesture may also refer to motor behavior that replaces speech (pantomime), and it is this meaing that is emphasized here. These nonverbal behaviors may be subdivided into several categories: (1) Iconic gestures express the meaning of the referent by the form of the gesture (e.g., moving the hand from a table to the mouth and back again to represent "eat "); (2) symbolic gestures bear an arbitrary relationship to their referents (e.g., forming the peak of a cap with the hand at the forehead to represent "boy"); and (3) indicative gestures represent the function of objects through the action performed (e.g., pretending to use a hammer). Two helpful review articles for an expanded version of gesture recognition for the interested reader are Peterson and Kirshner (1981) and Feyereisen and Seron (1982).

Speech is often accompanied by gesture, and the gestures may help a person to decode a message. For normal subjects this information may be redundant, but it may be an important ingredient to understanding for aphasic patients (Beukelman, Yorkston, and Waugh, 1980). Gesture is usually less impaired as a modality in aphasia (Porch, 1967) and therefore may be a profitable modality for treatment, particularly in those aphasic patients who have severe difficulties with other modalities.

As might be expected, studies that have investigated gesture recognition have generally used severe global aphasic individuals as their subjects (Varney, 1978; Peterson and Kirshner, 1981) because less severely impaired subjects are generally able to decode verbal language. Even in this restricted group, however, it has been difficult to predict which subjects to select for gestural training and which subjects will benefit from training.

Aphasic patients as a group are impaired in pantomime recognition when their performance is compared to normal controls (Duffy and Duffy, 1981; Duffy, Duffy, and Pearson, 1975; Feyereisen and Seron, 1982; Gainotti and Lemmo, 1976; Goodglass and Kaplan, 1963; Peterson and Kirshner, 1981; Varney, 1978, 1982). Defective performance is generally found in fewer than half the subjects tested (Varney, 1978, 1982), and the degree of deficit among defective performers is highly variable. Pantomime recognition performance correlates most highly with linguistic performance, rather than motor performance or intellectual performance (Duffy and Duffy, 1981; Varney, 1982), and more specifically with reading as opposed to other linguistic modalities or abilities (Varney, 1978, 1982).

Since gesture is reported to be less impaired in aphasia than verbal and graphic modalities and since some aphasic patients are not able to handle verbal language, gesture may serve as an alternate mode of communication. This possibility will be outlined in detail in the following chapter. A review of several articles in which Amer-Ind and/or ASL or pantomime have been employed and the outcome of such training are provided by Peterson and Kirschner (1981).

Stimuli. Whether an aphasic patient has difficulty recognizing a gesture appears to be related to several parameters of the test situation. Recognition of propositional gestures used to convey meaning (pantomime recognition) is impaired in many aphasic patients, whereas recognition of subpropositional gestures (facial expression) remains intact (Duffy and Buck, 1979). The nature of the response choices have been important to performance, with a hierarchy of response categories from easiest to most difficult listed below (Daniloff, Noll, Fristoe, and Lloyd, 1982; Netsu and Marquardt, 1984).

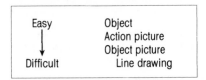

In addition, response choice relatedness has reportedly been an influence on performance in several studies. When the response array includes an item related to the target (correct) response, aphasic patients show a bias toward selecting the related item as opposed to unrelated foils (Daniloff et al., 1982; Duffy and Watkins, 1984; Varney and Benton, 1982). If the array contains an item with a similar plausible gesture to the target, this may also be a source of confusion for aphasic patients (Seron, van der Kaa, Remitz, and van der Linden, 1979).

Although gestures vary in their degree of relatedness to the object or action they represent, degree of symbolism was not a significant factor in gesture recognition (Duffy and McEwen, 1978). Therefore, success on a recognition task is difficult to predict on the basis of whether iconic or symbolic gestures are involved. Severity of aphasia does not appear to be related to gestural recognition performance (Daniloff et al., 1982). This would suggest that clinical success with gestural communication cannot be predicted from a patient's clinical severity but is more closely related to reading comprehension performance.

Description. These tasks are designed to work with understanding gestures, either singly or in series. The type of gesture or the gesture system employed might involve iconic, symbolic, or a combination of gesture types. These tasks are generally used with aphasic patients who are not comprehending the spoken word.

Example. In response to the clinician's gesture of whether the patient would like the window to be closed, the aphasic patient nods appropriately.

Area 5: Recognition of Spelling

Stimuli. Recognition of spelling is an area that requires visual processing as well as orthographic knowledge and graphemic-phonemic correspondences. In practical terms, its use is most frequently called upon in writing and proofreading tasks in which a decision has to be made regarding whether a word is spelled correctly. It may also be invoked when one is trying to decipher the meaning of the writing of a poor speller (e.g., *fone* for *phone*).

Recognition of spelling can be impaired in various types of aphasia (e.g., global, Broca's, Wernicke's) and in certain nonaphasic syndromes such as alexia with agraphia (Benson and Geschwind, 1969; Friedman, 1981; Patterson and Marcel, 1977).

The stimuli and tasks that researchers have used frequently fall into the categories of lexical decision tasks in which the aphasic individual (like the proofreader) is required to decide whether a particular string of letters is a word or a nonword. When aphasic patients are provided with real words and unrelated letter strings (nonwords, e.g., *dbxc*), they are able to make the distinction about which are words and which are not (Friedman, 1981). As Friedman pointed out, this decision can be based on the familiarity principle (Have I seen this word before?), orthographic regularity (Does this letter string correspond to the orthographic rules of English?), or both. When orthographically regular nonwords (pseudowords, e.g., *felp*) were to be separated from unrelated letter strings (e.g., *bdxc*), aphasics were relatively accurate in their decisions (Friedman, 1981), suggesting they retained some principles of orthographic processing. However, when it came to deciding between real words and pseudowords, many aphasic patients had difficulty and were unable to apply the principle of familiarity mentioned above (Friedman, 1981). In a related task requiring a lexical decision, Patterson and Marcel (1977) had normal controls and aphasic patients make lexical decisions about words and nonwords. The latter were divided into two categories, those that sounded like real words when pronounced (homophonic nonwords, e.g., *toun, flore*) and those that did not sound like real words when pronounced (nonhomophonic nonwords, e.g., *widge, dake*). The aphasic subjects failed to show a difference in processing these two categories, unlike the normal subjects. This suggested that they were not phonologically coding as were the normal subjects.

Lexical decision skills are also used by aphasic patients in reading their own writing when they must decide whether a word is spelled correctly. Here, they must apply both types of knowledge, familiarity and orthographic.

Based on this information, the following hierarchy, from easy to difficult, would seem to apply in treatment activities.

Easy	Category	Example
↓	Real word–unrelated letter string	cake–krty
	Pseudoword–unrelated letter string	dake–krty
	Real word–nonhomophonic nonword	cake–dake
Difficult	Real word–homophonic nonword	cake–kake

When recognition of spelling is fairly well retained, the errors that do occur accumulate on the final letters (Gardner and Zurif, 1976).

Description. Tasks in this area are designed to assist aphasic patients with recognition of correct spelling of their own or others' written language. The words may occur in isolation or in the context of longer material, such as sentences, paragraphs, essays, and so on.

Example. The aphasic patient is given his or her written narrative description of a picture and asked to locate, by underlining, any incorrectly spelled words.

Area 6: Reading Comprehension

Stimuli. In the area of reading comprehension the stimuli can occur as single words, phrases, sentences, or paragraphs. In general, as the length of material increases aphasic patients have more difficulty (Schuell et al., 1964; Van Demark et al., 1982; Wapner and Gardner, 1981) with comprehension. Therefore, the stimuli are arranged hierarchically.

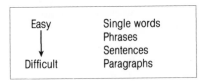

Easy	Single words
↓	Phrases
	Sentences
Difficult	Paragraphs

At each of these levels, various stimulus parameters can influence aphasic patients' performance. Frequency of occurrence is a potent variable, as is word length. The selection array from which the aphasic patient picks the response is also influential, with a rank order from easiest to hardest of auditory, semantic, and visual confusions (Gardner and Zurif, 1976; Van Demark et al., 1982).

For those aphasic individuals who adopt an analytical approach to reading by spelling a word letter by letter, using grapheme to phoneme conversion rules, the length of the word will significantly affect their performance. Locke and Deck (1982) reported that when aphasic patients were asked to cancel letters, such as *c, g,* and *h,* that occurred in words in sentence contexts, they made more errors on modal than nonmodal words. Modal words were those in which the letter was realized with a phonetic counterpart (e.g., *c* as /s/). Nonmodal words were those in which the letter did not have a direct phonetic counterpart (e.g., *c* in ch/tʃ/) or was silent (e.g., *h* as in "dou*g*h"). This suggested that the aphasic subjects were phonologically processing the words and were using grapheme to phoneme conversion rules. However, they did not have to comprehend the words to perform the task. Contrary to normal subjects, aphasic subjects did not show differential processing on this task for content and function words. This suggested that they did not process syntactic words differently as do normal individuals.

Comprehension of words was not significantly influenced by whether the stimulus to be matched was a picture or a printed word. However, whether the selection choices were acoustically or semantically related to the target did affect performance (Gardner and Zurif, 1976).

Easy	Stimulus	Response Array
	One picture	Four acoustically related words
	One word	Four acoustically related pictures
	One picture	Four semantically related pictures
Difficult	One word	Four semantically related words

Other features that affect single word comprehension are operativity, figurativity (referents that are not easily manipulated by touch), abstractness of nouns, and grammatical form class. Since severity of aphasia affected these results, hierarchies are shown for groups with mild and significant comprehension deficits (Gardner and Zurif, 1976).

Easy	Mild Comprehension Deficit	Example	Significant Comprehension Deficit
	Operative noun	Book	Operative noun
	Figurative noun	Ocean	Mixed parts of speech
	Abstract noun	Hope	Figurative noun
	Verb	Wash	Abstract noun
Difficult	Mixed parts of speech		Verb

Paradigmatic associations are slightly easier than syntagmatic ones although the differences were not statistically significant (Gardner and Zurif, 1976).

For phrase material, length, grammatical form class, composition, and the amount of content words relative to overall length have been influential for reading comprehension. Although type of aphasia was not a significant contributor to differential performance, severity of comprehension deficit was. The hierarchy reported by Gardner and Zurif (1976) follows.

Easy	Length	Construction	Example
	Long	Head Noun–Progressive–Noun	The small happy boy watching the speeding silver airplane
	Brief	Noun–Progressive	Dog eating
	Long	Noun–Progressive	The black and white puppy dog eating the dirty brown shoe
	Brief	Progressive–Noun	Watching airplane
	Brief	Noun–Preposition–Noun	Shoes on rug
Difficult	Long	Noun–Preposition–Noun	New black shoes lying on the soft blue rug

Therefore, preposition constructions were difficult for the aphasic subjects. The lengthy versions of the constructions were easier for patients with mild aphasia, provided that increasing length added a substantive word, thereby increasing content. Severely impaired aphasic patients found the lengthy items more difficult.

Wapner and Gardner (1981) found performance deficits in Broca's and Wernicke's aphasic subjects for phrase comprehension. The Broca's errors showed a trend toward selecting a syntactically anomalous phrase, such as "write pencil," rather than one more similar to the target. This is consistent with other reports of syntactic processing deficits in Broca's aphasia.

The research literature generally reveals that aphasic patients have difficulty understanding written sentences. This is not surprising in view of the material presented previously demonstrating word and phrase reading comprehension deficits. Some studies have provided additional information about the kinds of sentences that are more difficult and the kinds of errors that different groups of aphasic patients make. This information is helpful in designing therapy, because it allows the clinician to use sentence material at an appropriate level and of appropriate content to emphasize certain features, semantically or syntactically.

Easy	**Anterior Lesion Patients**	**Example**	**Posterior Lesions Patients**	
	SAAD (nonreversible)[1]	The boy ate the sandwich.	SAAD (nonreversible)	
	True/False		True/False	Fill in Blank
	Semantic	An inch is a unit of weight.	Semantic =	Semantic =
	Syntactic	Five follows three.	Syntactic	Syntactic
	Fill in Blank			
	Semantic	A machine that flies is called a _____.		
	Syntactic	A nickel is worth _____. than a dime.		
Difficult	SAAD (reversible)	The boy pushed the girl.		

[1] SAAD refers to simple active affirmative declarative sentences.

These hierarchies are based on results reported by von Stockert and Bader (1976), Samuels and Benson (1979), Caramazza, Berndt, Basili, and Koller (1981) and Gallaher and Canter (1982).

Gardner, Denes, and Zurif (1975) found similar results for the semantic versus syntactic sentence comprehension hierarchy and no differences between anterior and posterior aphasic groups. Since their materials were somewhat different from the previous studies, the separate hierarchies are shown for semantically anomalous and syntactically deviant sentences.

Easy	Semantic Hierarchy	Example
↓	Erroneous proper noun	The President lives in **Boston**.
	Subject-object reversal	The **milk** drank the **cat**.
	Transitive sentence with anomalous verb	The dog **seemed** the cat.
	Incorrect number	The week has **six** days.
	Erroneous adjective	Birds fly in the **green** sky.
	Anomalous noun as object	John drives his new **road**.
	Erroneous verb	The boy **ate** his milk.
Difficult	Incorrect passive	The dog was bitten by the man.

Easy	Syntactic Hierarchies Anterior Lesion Patients	Posterior Lesion Patients		Example
↓	Incorrect case	Number	Case	John sat on **him** chair.
	Incorrect gender	Gender	Gender	The girl raised **his** arms.
	Incorrect verb form	Case	Verb form	He **giving** the cat milk.
	Incorrect article	Word order	Article	She gave John **the** kiss.
	Incorrect number	Article	Number	The dog lifted **their** legs.
Difficult	Incorrect word order	Verb	Word order	Give me **red three** apples.

Beyond SAAD sentences, investigators have found that certain sentence types are more difficult to comprehend than others. It has been found that Broca's and conduction aphasic groups have particular difficulty with syntactic processing, whereas the same significant syntactic factor was not evident for Wernike's aphasic patients (Caramazza et al., 1981; Rothi, McFarling, and Heilman, 1982). Whether sentences correspond to a picture–real life situation and whether the task presented is one of reading comprehension or written sentence formulation from constituent sentence parts, have also played roles in reading comprehension. When the sentence is presented in segments divided at constituent boundaries, sentence formulation can be more difficult than when the constituents are contained within the segments. The following hierarchies are condensed from the work of Levy and Taylor (1968), Deloche and Seron (1981), and von Stockert (1972).

Easy	Sentence Type	Picture Match Truth Value	Correspond to World Knowledge	Sentence Construction Segments	Example
	SAAD Active	True	Yes	(N) Nonconstituent parts	This /car uses lots/ of oil.
		False	No	(C) Constituent parts	This car /uses/ diesel oil.
			Irrelevant		This car is red.
	Negative-Passive	False	—	—	The letter was not typed by the secretary.
		True			The letter was not typed by the baby.
	Passive	True, false	—	—	The window was broken by the ball.
	Negative	False	—	—	It is not cold in December.
		True	—		It is not hot in December.
	Embedded sentences	—	—	NC, C	The man who is wearing a hat is a policeman.
	Questions	—	—	NC, C	Where is the car?
Difficult	Imperatives	—	—	NC, C	Close the door.

Length of the sentence can be an important variable to control although increased length may not affect different types of aphasia in the same way. Length generally reduces reading comprehension in Broca's aphasia whereas Wernicke's aphasic patients may do better with the additional context and added redundancy (Albert et al., 1981; Schuell et al., 1964).

Aphasic patients' performance on paragraph comprehension of aphasia test batteries and clinical reports show that paragraphs are more difficult stimuli than sentences. The parameters that seem to be important contributors to comprehension at this level are length of the paragraph and individual sentences within it, thematic content, vocabulary, syntactic complexity of the sentences, and so forth. General measures such as grade level or readability, as measured by a variety of formulae, can also be used to arrange paragraphs according to difficulty level. Therefore, treatment materials can be selected from sources of materials arranged by grade level.

Variables to Control
Length
    Overall
    Sentences
Content
Vocabulary
    Frequency of occurrence
Syntactic complexity

The variables to control in contructing stimuli are the aforementioned. As a general rule of thumb, only one variable should be increased at a time to avoid making the material too difficult. Of course, for rapidly advancing advancing patients this can be altered to permit the patient to progress as quickly as possible.

Responding to questions has been a traditional way to evaluate reading comprehension. Patients tend to score higher on factual questions compared with inferential questions.

Some sources for readability formulae can be found in Appendix 4-1.

Description. Activities within this area are designed to improve the aphasic patient's understanding of linguistic units. As these units are gradually increased in complexity, the aphasic individual comprehends more difficult material. At higher levels of functioning, activities may include drawing inferences from reading passages as well as factual questions.

Example. The aphasic patient reads a sentence silently and then matches it with its corresponding picture, selecting from an array of three. The choices represent the correct picture, the reverse of the agent-object, and the same agent-object performing a different action.

Area 7: Reading Textual Material

Stimuli. The stimuli for reading passages in this area actually represent an extension of paragraphs described in Area 6. Although many aphasic patients recover to the extent that they can manage paragraphs, many are not able to resume regular reading activity levels. These may deal with longer material and higher difficulty levels found in technical reports, business reports and correspondence, and so on. Reportedly, even though aphasic patients can improve to cope with more complex material, they no longer find reading pleasurable; it is a slow and laborious task (Kaplan and Goodglass, 1981). Although the majority of patients may not read complex material, it is an important area for some, particularly those who may return to the workforce in a position that requires reading at this level.

The following stimuli are not hierarchically arranged. Within each type of material, difficulty can be increased by altering the variables listed after the stimuli.

Short stories
Magazine articles
Newspaper articles and editorials
Business and advertising letters
Journal material
Reports
        Business, technical, agency

Novels
Essays

Variables to Control
Length
General complexity
    Grade level
      Readability level
Vocabulary
Redundancy
Grammatical complexity
Cohesion
Anaphoric reference
Familiarity of topic

Description. From the stimuli involved, it is apparent that the activities for this area represent an advanced level of performance. They are designed to encourage the aphasic patient to comprehend material encountered in many daily life situations. Since they are at a high level, they are directed to those people who premorbidly read complex material, who read extensively for pleasure, or both. The materials increase, in general, in length and complexity.

Example. The aphasic patient reads a technical report (e.g., how to increase crop output or the financial benefits of deferred income) and abstracts four or five key points made by the author.

APPENDIX 4–1

SOURCES FOR READABILITY FORMULAE

Elementary Level

Fry, E. B. (1968). A readability formula that saves time. *Journal of Reading, 11,* 513–516, 575–578.

Spache, G. D. (1978). *Good reading for poor readers* (185–197). Champaign, IL: Garrad.

Fourth, Fifth Grade to College

Chall, D. E., and Chall, J. (1948). A formula for predicting readability. *Educational Research Bulletin, 27,* 11–20.

Chall, D. E., and Chall, J. (1948). A formula for predicting readability: Instructions. *Educational Research Bulletin, 27,* 37–54.

Flesch, R. (1951). *How to test readability.* New York: Harper and Row.

Secondary to Adult

Gunning, R. (1968). *The technique of clear writing* (37–39). New York: McGraw-Hill.

McLaughlin, G. (1969). SMOG Grading—A new readability formula. *Journal of Reading, 12,* 639–646.

Chapter 5

Materials for Visual Processing

Area 1: Matching Nonverbal Material

Beginning Levels

Level 1

Stimuli. Pairs of identical familiar objects

Set A		Set B	
1.	pencil	1.	cup
2.	paper clip	2.	fork
3.	paper	3.	spoon
4.	eraser	4.	knife
5.	pin	5.	saucer
6.	key	6.	glass
7.	quarter	7.	bowl
8.	sock	8.	napkin
9.	earring	9.	napkin ring
10.	shoelace	10.	plate

Procedure. The following sets of objects are placed in front of the patient. The clinician presents the replica of the underlined word, and the patient points to the appropriate matching object.

Set A

1.	pencil	key	bowl
2.	cup	paper clip	earring
3.	eraser	paper	spoon
4.	plate	socks	eraser
5.	spoon	pin	fork
6.	key	napkin ring	shoelace
7.	quarter	saucer	knife
8.	quarter	glass	sock
9.	napkin	earring	bowl
10.	key	spoon	shoelace

Set B

1.	pencil	cup	plate
2.	napkin	fork	paper clip
3.	earring	bowl	spoon
4.	knife	napkin ring	eraser
5.	spoon	saucer	shoelace
6.	glass	paper	fork
7.	cup	sock	bowl
8.	quarter	glass	napkin
9.	napkin ring	key	saucer
10.	pen	plate	knife

Level 2

Stimuli. Objects, along with pictured representations

Set A		Set B	
1.	book	1.	razor
2.	comb	2.	ball
3.	watch	3.	screwdriver
4.	box	4.	clock
5.	doll	5.	saw
6.	eggbeater	6.	telephone
7.	pencil	7.	ring
8.	pitcher	8.	hanger
9.	brush	9.	purse
10.	shoe	10.	hammer

Procedure. The following sets of three pictured objects are placed in front of the patient. The clinician presents the object representing the underlined word, and the patient places it on or points to the corresponding picture.

Set A

1.	book	razor	shoe
2.	comb	hammer	ring
3.	purse	ball	watch
4.	box	hanger	telephone
5.	screwdriver	doll	clock
6.	eggbeater	saw	comb
7.	razor	purse	pencil
8.	clock	watch	pitcher
9.	doll	brush	saw
10.	screwdriver	shoe	telephone

Set B

1.	book	ring	razor
2.	hanger	ball	comb
3.	screwdriver	watch	box
4.	clock	doll	brush
5.	purse	saw	ball
6.	hammer	telephone	book
7.	eggbeater	screwdriver	ring
8.	pencil	box	hanger
9.	saw	brush	purse
10.	hammer	pitcher	ball

Level 3

Stimuli. Nonidentical pairs of pictures representing the same objects: for example, two different styles of chair

Set A

1. tree
2. chair
3. coat
4. bed
5. car
6. dog
7. house
8. airplane
9. television
10. lamp

Set B

1. table
2. bird
3. train
4. radio
5. dress
6. flower
7. apple
8. shirt
9. boat
10. hat

Procedure. The following sets of pictures are placed in front of the patient. The clinician presents the alternate pictured representation of the underlined word, and the patient points to the appropriate picture.

Set A

1.	lamp	tree	table
2.	chair	bird	dress
3.	train	airplane	coat
4.	radio	house	bed
5.	dress	car	radio
6.	dog	television	chair
7.	house	apple	shirt
8.	airplane	table	hat
9.	tree	television	flower
10.	boat	bird	lamp

Set B

1.	coat	hat	table
2.	boat	car	bird
3.	bed	flower	train
4.	radio	apple	shirt
5.	dress	house	airplane
6.	television	flower	lamp
7.	hat	dog	apple
8.	shirt	radio	chair
9.	dress	boat	tree
10.	apple	hat	flower

Additional Levels

Additional levels may be developed by altering the number and kind of choices available to the patient. The task could be made more difficult, for example, by presenting choices from the same semantic category. The categories of colors, forms, and actions could also be included.

Area 2: Matching Verbal Material

Beginning Levels

Level 1

Stimuli. Printed three-letter words; visually dissimilar choices

Set A		Set B	
1.	war	1.	hat
2.	put	2.	top
3.	leg	3.	get
4.	car	4.	ear
5.	big	5.	kit
6.	two	6.	dog
7.	son	7.	van
8.	met	8.	red
9.	far	9.	jar
10.	new	10.	lot

Procedure. The following sets of three printed words are placed in front of the patient. The clinician presents a card with the underlined word printed on it, and the patient points to the matching word in the series.

Set A

1.	<u>war</u>	pen	hit
2.	dad	bee	<u>put</u>
3.	nut	cap	<u>leg</u>
4.	zoo	<u>car</u>	tip
5.	rob	<u>big</u>	tax
6.	bet	lap	<u>two</u>
7.	<u>son</u>	rub	wet
8.	lad	<u>met</u>	sin
9.	<u>far</u>	nod	gem
10.	<u>new</u>	toe	pad

Set B

1.	tee	<u>hat</u>	wed
2.	<u>top</u>	sew	mat
3.	eat	pen	<u>get</u>
4.	fat	lad	<u>ear</u>
5.	own	<u>kit</u>	man
6.	<u>dog</u>	can	rat
7.	<u>van</u>	boy	jam
8.	bat	age	<u>red</u>
9.	buy	<u>jar</u>	tin
10.	yes	pay	<u>lot</u>

Level 2

Stimuli. Printed three-letter words; visually similar choices

Set A		Set B	
1.	dam	1.	gum
2.	bug	2.	ore
3.	sap	3.	pad
4.	rim	4.	hem
5.	cab	5.	jaw
6.	not	6.	lid
7.	fog	7.	vat
8.	eat	8.	age
9.	tam	9.	nip
10.	keg	10.	mat

Procedure. The following sets of three printed words are placed in front of the patient. The clinician presents a card with the underlined word printed on it, and the patient points to the matching word in the series.

Set A

1.	<u>dam</u>	ham	dim
2.	big	<u>bug</u>	dug
3.	sad	sop	<u>sap</u>
4.	ram	run	<u>rim</u>
5.	cap	<u>cab</u>	cub
6.	<u>not</u>	net	nut
7.	<u>fog</u>	fig	log
8.	oat	ear	<u>eat</u>
9.	tan	<u>tam</u>	tim
10.	peg	<u>keg</u>	key

Set B

1.	gun	<u>gum</u>	gem
2.	are	<u>ore</u>	ode
3.	pat	pod	<u>pad</u>
4.	<u>hem</u>	hew	hen
5.	paw	<u>jaw</u>	jar
6.	lad	lip	<u>lid</u>
7.	vet	van	<u>vat</u>
8.	ape	ago	<u>age</u>
9.	<u>nip</u>	nap	hip
10.	<u>mat</u>	met	map

Level 3

Stimuli. Printed two-word phrases; seven letters; visually dissimilar choices

Set A		Set B	
1.	you came	1.	mad boss
2.	sit down	2.	war game
3.	try some	3.	get lost
4.	eat more	4.	pay rent
5.	hit hard	5.	not less
6.	new coat	6.	ten pins
7.	hot milk	7.	sad time
8.	big room	8.	had they
9.	one hour	9.	bad shot
10.	ask them	10.	wet hair

Procedure. Two printed phrases are placed in front of the patient. The clinician provides the underlined words printed on a card, and the patient matches them to the appropriate phrase.

Set A

1.	you came	cry wolf
2.	sit down	leg cast
3.	try some	mud pies
4.	you lose	eat more
5.	dad went	hit hard
6.	new coat	lap tray
7.	any word	hot milk
8.	tin cans	big room
9.	one hour	not true
10.	tree top	ask them

Set B

1.	two feet	mad boss
2.	dog gone	old game
3.	get lost	ear full
4.	pay rent	use ours
5.	red rose	not less
6.	tin pins	car load
7.	eye sore	sad time
8.	old news	had they
9.	bad shot	tax tips
10.	ice cold	wet hair

Additional Levels

Additional levels can be developed by altering the length of the stimuli, by providing visually similar printed choices, or by removing the printed stimulus, prior to the patient's response.

Area 3: Visual Correspondence/Recognition

1. Association of Visual Materials

Beginning Levels

Level 1

Stimuli. Letters of the alphabet, capitalized and noncapitalized

Procedure. The following sets of printed letters are placed in front of the patient. A capital letter corresponding to one of the letters in the series is presented and the patient points to the appropriate item.

Set A

1.	D	j	d	c	z
2.	F:	o	g	n	f
3.	R:	r	e	w	p
4.	B:	a	l	s	b
5.	L:	b	u	x	l
6.	T:	p	t	m	a
7.	C:	c	h	y	k
8.	N:	d	n	s	q
9.	V:	v	e	l	p
10.	O:	z	f	j	o

Set B

1.	A:	a	v	s	b
2.	W:	l	d	e	w
3.	U:	r	k	u	f
4.	K:	k	g	i	x
5.	Z:	c	z	h	n
6.	E:	j	p	r	e
7.	G:	g	f	k	m
8.	X:	o	l	x	n
9.	H:	m	h	p	z
10.	M:	m	q	y	i

Level 2

Stimuli. Printed four-letter strings: nonwords and real words

Procedure. The following four-letter strings are placed in front of the patient. The patient is required to point to the real word.

Set A

1. race	btro	kgoe
2. vrtp	loss	nvwm
3. foot	sbta	urqw
4. date	eldp	nmoe
5. bdqc	cold	kzci
6. okdr	tcue	love
7. hdae	ivzr	send
8. rnel	pass	wrcd
9. turn	nvak	hrez
10. pdra	lwpo	door

Set B

1. look	wmra	zuei
2. tldi	euai	game
3. nhkl	vote	dpro
4. salt	qvae	bcri
5. tldb	akmr	ship
6. they	jxvb	gdzo
7. ulba	farm	npbe
8. fhke	ldro	bird
9. room	sxzi	awhk
10. fgnp	tboa	spot

Level 3

Stimuli. Printed four-letter strings: nonwords (*txrn*), real words (*boat*), and pseudowords (*naib*)

Procedure. The following four-letter strings are placed in front of the patient. The patient is required to point to the real word.

Set A

1. pain	hain	rtpx
2. kztr	zost	most
3. mamp	camp	ltap
4. reat	seat	vnel
5. lose	ekcd	sose
6. kath	lnzo	path
7. ldpu	gone	fone
8. wait	hait	sdei
9. zeat	heat	xvwi
10. pdec	race	nace

Set B

1.	mnuv	pree	<u>tree</u>
2.	leat	<u>meat</u>	uenk
3.	<u>will</u>	cill	rdou
4.	zpea	<u>sing</u>	hing
5.	hish	<u>fish</u>	ldpa
6.	yose	adbp	<u>nose</u>
7.	nast	vwor	<u>last</u>
8.	<u>kiss</u>	wiss	nsta
9.	nade	<u>made</u>	eqap
10.	jull	tcak	<u>pull</u>

Association of Visual Materials: Additional Levels

Additional levels may be developed by including more visually similar choices in the response array.

2.   Association of Materials Within a Superordinate Category

Beginning Levels

Level 1

Stimuli. Sets of pictured nouns belonging to the same category

Set A

	Kitchen Utensils	**Clothing**	**Toys**
1.	knife	shirt	doll
2.	spoon	socks	ball
3.	fork	pants	rattle
4.	pan	coat	gun
5.	pot	dress	rocking horse
6.	spatula	hat	doll buggy
7.	can opener	sweater	game
8.	stove	tie	block
9.	bowl	slip	boat
10.	mixer	jacket	top

Set B

	Furniture	**Musical Instruments**	**Vehicles**
1.	chair	piano	car
2.	table	drum	bus
3.	bed	trumpet	airplane
4.	sofa	violin	train

5.	desk	cello	truck
6.	lamp	flute	bicycle
7.	dresser	guitar	motorcycle
8.	television	accordion	boat
9.	stool	trombone	scooter
10.	rug	tuba	wagon

Procedure. Thirty pictures are placed in front of the patient to sort into three unrelated categories, each consisting of 10 members.

Level 2

Stimuli. A set of pictured nouns belonging to the same category

Set A: Animals

Domestic		**Wild**	
1.	cat	1.	bear
2.	calf	2.	beaver
3.	dog	3.	buffalo
4.	duck	4.	camel
5.	goat	5.	dinosaur
6.	goose	6.	giraffe
7.	hen	7.	hippopotamus
8.	horse	8.	leopard
9.	pig	9.	lion
10.	sheep	10.	moose

Set B: Food

Fruit		**Vegetables**	
1.	apple	1.	carrot
2.	orange	2.	pea
3.	pear	3.	corn
4.	banana	4.	bean
5.	peach	5.	potato
6.	grape	6.	cauliflower
7.	cherry	7.	lettuce
8.	plum	8.	spinach
9.	grapefruit	9.	asparagus
10.	lemon	10.	broccoli

Procedure. Twenty pictures of the same semantic category are placed in front of the patient to sort into two subcategories.

Level 3

Stimuli. Pairs of semantically related pictured nouns

Set A

1. paper/pen: easel/paintbrush
2. carton/milk: can/soup
3. hammer/nail: screwdriver/screw
4. bat/ball: hockey stick/puck
5. teeth/toothbrush: face/washcloth
6. bird/nest: bee/hive
7. chef/kitchen: secretary/office
8. doctor/stethoscope: dentist/drill
9. suitcase/clothes: wallet/money
10. shovel/snow: rake/leaves

Set B

1. sock/foot: glove/hand
2. picture/wall: rug/floor
3. mechanic/car: veterinarian/animal
4. book/magazine: glass/cup
5. bread/toaster: water/kettle
6. door/gate: bathtub/sink
7. orange/grapefruit: apple/pear
8. pants/belt: shoes/shoelaces
9. car/bus: helicopter/airplane
10. knife/meat: spoon/cereal

Procedure. A pair of pictures is placed in front of the patient. A third picture is presented, and the patient must choose from an array of three one which demonstrates an analogous relationship.

Set A

1. paper/pen: easel/
   <u>paintbrush</u>   pencil   paint
2. carton/milk: can/
   can opener   bananas   <u>soup</u>
3. hammer/nail: screwdriver/
   <u>screw</u>   saw   wrench
4. bat/ball: hockey stick/
   <u>puck</u>   hockey net   skates
5. teeth/toothbrush: face/
   towel   <u>washcloth</u>   soap

6. bird/nest: bee/
   flower   honey   <u>hive</u>
7. chef/kitchen: secretary/
   farm   <u>office</u>   typewriter
8. doctor/stethoscope: dentist/
   toothbrush   <u>drill</u>   patient
9. suitcase/clothes: wallet/
   purse   <u>money</u>   bank
10. shovel/snow: rake/
    <u>leaves</u>   flowers   beach

Set B

1. sock/foot: glove/
   <u>hand</u>   hat   church
2. picture/wall: rug/
   <u>floor</u>   vacuum cleaner   living room
3. mechanic/car: veterinarian/
   barn   <u>animal</u>   stethoscope
4. book/magazine: glass/
   <u>cup</u>   water   window
5. bread/toaster: water/
   pitcher   sink   <u>kettle</u>
6. door/gate: bathtub/
   bathroom   <u>sink</u>   soap
7. orange/grapefruit: apple/
   cake   <u>pear</u>   pie
8. pants/belt: shoes/
   <u>shoelaces</u>   brush   socks
9. car/bus: helicopter/
   pilot   boat   <u>airplane</u>
10. knife/meat: spoon/
    bowl   <u>cereal</u>   fork

Area 4: Reception of Gestured Messages

Beginning Levels

Level 1

Stimuli. Real objects

Set A	Set B
1. cup	1. knife
2. pen	2. comb
3. paintbrush	3. whisk
4. saw	4. razor
5. spoon	5. towel
6. toothbrush	6. pitcher
7. pipe	7. fly swatter
8. screwdriver	8. nail file
9. telephone	9. lipstick
10. calculator	10. perfume

Procedure. Three objects are placed in front of the patient. The clinician gestures the function of the underlined word, and the patient points to the corresponding item.

Set A

1. cup	perfume	calculator
2. telephone	pen	pitcher
3. pipe	paintbrush	towel
4. saw	toothbrush	lipstick
5. fly swatter	nail file	spoon
6. screwdriver	toothbrush	knife
7. pipe	comb	whisk
8. cup	razor	screwdriver
9. saw	pen	telephone
10. spoon	paintbrush	calculator

Set B

1. calculator	knife	lipstick
2. nail file	pipe	comb
3. whisk	toothbrush	saw
4. razor	spoon	paintbrush
5. pen	towel	cup
6. toothbrush	perfume	pitcher
7. fly swatter	calculator	knife
8. cup	nail file	pipe
9. lipstick	pitcher	pen
10. screwdriver	telephone	perfume

Level 2

Stimuli. Action pictures

Set A

1. eating
2. combing hair
3. setting a table
4. sharpening a pencil
5. telephoning
6. writing
7. driving
8. hammering
9. knocking at a door
10. washing hands

Set A

1. drinking
2. sawing
3. painting
4. opening a window
5. fighting
6. swimming
7. throwing
8. playing a piano
9. clapping
10. shaving

Procedure. Three action pictures are placed in front of the patient. The clinician performs the action corresponding to the underlined word, and the patient points to the corresponding picture.

Set A

1. eating	sawing	knocking at a door
2. painting	washing hands	combing hair
3. hammering	drinking	setting a table
4. fighting	sharpening a pencil	opening a window
5. telephoning	driving	swimming
6. throwing	writing	shaving
7. eating	playing a piano	driving
8. clapping	hammering	telephoning
9. combing hair	knocking at a door	writing
10. washing hands	setting a table	sharpening a pencil

Set B

1. shaving	drinking	combing hair
2. knocking at a door	eating	sawing
3. clapping	telephoning	painting
4. opening a window	playing a piano	throwing
5. fighting	writing	hammering
6. drinking	swimming	sharpening a pencil
7. setting a table	washing hands	throwing
8. playing a piano	fighting	washing hands
9. clapping	swimming	painting
10. opening a window	driving	shaving

Level 3

Stimuli. Line drawings of objects

Set A		Set B	
1.	cup	1.	knife
2.	pen	2.	comb
3.	paintbrush	3.	whisk
4.	saw	4.	razor
5.	spoon	5.	towel
6.	toothbrush	6.	pitcher
7.	pipe	7.	fly swatter
8.	screwdriver	8.	nail file
9.	telephone	9.	lipstick
10.	calculator	10.	perfume

Procedure. Three line drawings of objects are placed in front of the patient. The clinician gestures the function of the underlined word, and the patient points to the corresponding drawing.

Set A

1.	calculator	perfume	cup
2.	telephone	razor	pen
3.	paintbrush	comb	knife
4.	pipe	saw	toothbrush
5.	perfume	towel	spoon
6.	nail file	toothbrush	fly swatter
7.	pipe	cup	pen
8.	pitcher	screwdriver	lipstick
9.	telephone	spoon	saw
10.	paintbrush	whisk	calculator

Set B

1.	knife	perfume	fly swatter
2.	comb	screwdriver	pitcher
3.	nail file	whisk	calculator
4.	telephone	razor	pipe
5.	saw	pen	towel
6.	pitcher	spoon	paintbrush
7.	screwdriver	fly swatter	towel
8.	comb	cup	nail file
9.	razor	lipstick	knife
10.	towel	whisk	perfume

Additional Levels

Additional levels might be developed by selecting related items, as opposed to unrelated items for foils. Including items in the array with similar plausible gestures to the targets may make the task more difficult. Also, two gestures may be combined for matching an appropriate item.

Area 5: Recognition of Spelling

The following material was designed for patients demonstrating surface dyslexia.

Beginning Levels

Level 1

Stimuli. Pairs of printed real words and homophonic nonwords; printed nouns

Set A	Set B
1. bird–berd	1. boat–bote
2. tree–trea	2. face–fase
3. door–dore	3. meat–mete
4. car–kar	4. knee–nee
5. feet–fete	5. coat–kote
6. game–gaim	6. house–howse
7. suit–sute	7. moon–mune
8. boy–boi	8. dog–dawg
9. nose–noze	9. box–bocks
10. shoe–shue	10. roof–rufe

Procedure. A picture is placed in front of the patient, along with a printed real word and a homophonic nonword. The patient points to the word corresponding to the picture.

Level 2

Stimuli. Pairs of printed real words and homonyms; pictured nouns, pronouns, verbs, and adjectives

Set A	Set B
1. bear–bare	1. wait–weight
2. feet–feat	2. sun–son
3. cent–sent	3. maid–made
4. meat–meet	4. cot–caught
5. eight–ate	5. sail–sale

6.	walk–wok	6.	beet–beat
7.	hair–hare	7.	rain–rein
8.	pear–pair	8.	steak–stake
9.	bee–be	9.	knot–not
10.	red–read	10.	tea–tee

Procedure. A picture is placed in front of the patient, along with a printed real word and a homonym. The patient points to the word corresponding to the picture.

Level 3

Stimuli. Sets of sentences: one with correct spelling, one containing a homophonic nonword, and one containing a homonym

Set A

1. a. The bear attacked the man.
    b. The bare attacked the man.
    c. The bair attacked the man.
2. a. My feat ache.
    b. My fete ache.
    c. My feet ache.
3. a. I didn't lose a cent.
    b. I didn't lose a sent.
    c. I didn't lose a centt.
4. a. She broiled the meat.
    b. She broiled the meet.
    c. She broiled the miete.
5. a. The boy saved ate dollars.
    b. The boy saved ait dollars.
    c. The boy saved eight dollars.
6. a. The children walk to school.
    b. The children wock to school.
    c. The children wok to school.
7. a. The barber cut his hare.
    b. The barber cut his hair.
    c. The barber cut his herr.
8. a. The pair is too ripe.
    b. The pare is too ripe.
    c. The pear is too ripe.
9. a. The girl was stung by the bea.
    b. The girl was stung by the bee.
    c. The girl was stung by the be.
10. a. The car went through the red light.
    b. The car went through the read light.
    c. The car went through the redd light.

Set B

1. a. We weight for the mail every morning.
   b. We wate for the mail every morning.
   c. We wait for the mail every morning.
2. a. His sun plays baseball.
   b. His son plays baseball.
   c. His scun plays baseball.
3. a. The maid wanted a raise.
   b. The mayd wanted a raise.
   c. The made wanted a raise.
4. a. The guest slept on a caught.
   b. The guest slept on a cot.
   c. The guest slept on a kot.
5. a. They sail every summer.
   b. They sale every summer.
   c. They sayl every summer.
6. a. The gardener planted beatts.
   b. The gardener planted beats.
   c. The gardener planted beets.
7. a. The rain damaged the crop.
   b. The rein damaged the crop.
   c. The rane damaged the crop.
8. a. The waiter served the stake.
   b. The waiter served the stache.
   c. The waiter served the steak.
9. a. The rope was tied in a not.
   b. The rope was tied in a nawt.
   c. The rope was tied in a knot.
10. a. Her husband poured the tea.
    b. Her husband poured the tee.
    c. Her husband poured the teah.

Procedure. Three printed sentences are placed in front of the patient. The patient selects the sentence with the correct spelling.

Area 6: Reading Comprehension

Beginning Levels

Level 1

Stimuli. Pictured nouns
Printed words: four letters long; grades 1 to 4 vocabulary

Set A	Set B
1. bird	1. room
2. door	2. leaf
3. game	3. star
4. tree	4. maid
5. lion	5. duck
6. horn	6. bell
7. vest	7. shoe
8. meat	8. rice
9. drum	9. seal
10. fork	10. neck

Procedure. The following sets of three pictured nouns are presented to the patient. The underlined printed word is presented, and the patient points to the picture it represents. The choices are acoustically and semantically unrelated.

Set A

1.	bird	chair	train
2.	coat	door	baby
3.	bed	game	dog
4.	foot	king	tree
5.	dress	lion	table
6.	horn	cup	gate
7.	bear	vest	saw
8.	meat	sun	leg
9.	rose	box	drum
10.	watch	fork	nose

Set B

1.	gun	cake	room
2.	ball	pen	leaf
3.	star	toy	dish
4.	flag	maid	cat
5.	skirt	van	duck
6.	mouse	belt	rain
7.	shoe	horse	milk
8.	rice	shirt	boat
9.	toast	hat	seal
10.	soup	neck	glove

Level 2

Stimuli. Pictured nouns and numbers
Printed words: four letters long; grades 1 to 4 vocabulary

Set A	Set B
1. book	1. rose
2. ring	2. moon
3. lake	3. seat
4. nose	4. cook
5. cent	5. fish
6. bear	6. coat
7. soap	7. sign
8. dish	8. king
9. door	9. cake
10. suit	10. boat

Procedure. The following sets of three pictured nouns are presented to the patient. The underlined printed word is presented, and the patient points to the picture it represents. One foil is a semantically related picture and another is an acoustically similar response.

Set A

1.	cook	book	magazine
2.	watch	ring	king
3.	lake	swimming pool	cake
4.	mouth	hose	nose
5.	dollar	cent	tent
6.	dog	hair	bear
7.	towel	rope	soap
8.	dish	fish	spoon
9.	door	four	window
10.	shirt	suit	soup

Set B

1.	rose	toes	tree
2.	moon	sun	spoon
3.	seat	feet	table
4.	pot	book	cook
5.	dish	bird	fish
6.	boat	coat	hat
7.	sign	line	picture
8.	queen	ring	king
9.	rake	cake	pie
10.	shop	ship	boat

Level 3

Stimuli. Pictured nouns

Printed two-word phrases: two to four syllables; grades 1 to 4 vocabulary

Set A		Set B	
1.	red coat	1.	busy man
2.	big house	2.	green circle
3.	clean clothes	3.	fat boy
4.	hot day	4.	many people
5.	black suit	5.	huge truck
6.	sad girl	6.	cold milk
7.	wide road	7.	sick child
8.	old car	8.	dirty face
9.	raw meat	9.	blue shirt
10.	pretty woman	10.	fresh fruit

Procedure. A pictured noun is placed in front of the patient, along with three printed phrases. The patient points to the phrase corresponding to the picture.

Set A

1.	red coat	blue coat	red shirt
2.	big hand	small house	big house
3.	clean cups	clean clothes	dirty clothes
4.	cold day	hot day	hot night
5.	black dress	white suit	black suit
6.	sad girl	happy girl	sad boy
7.	wide race	little road	wide road
8.	old boat	old car	new car
9.	raw meat	raw potato	white meat
10.	pretty girl	ugly woman	pretty woman

Set B

1.	busy man	busy boy	small man
2.	green city	green circle	red circle
3.	fat boy	thin boy	fat man
4.	many flowers	few people	many people
5.	huge truck	huge trunk	tiny truck
6.	hot milk	cold milk	cold meat
7.	sick child	sick baby	strong child
8.	dirty face	clean face	dirty feet
9.	blue shoe	black shirt	blue shirt
10.	fresh eggs	soft fruit	fresh fruit

Additional Levels

Additional levels may be developed by introducing sentences. Parameters to be varied might include vocabulary difficulty, length, and syntactic complexity.

Area 7: Reading Complex Material

Beginning Levels

Level 1

Stimuli. Short newspaper advertisements; true/false statements

Procedure. The patient reads a short newspaper advertisement. True/false statements about its content are provided in printed form or may be auditorily presented. The patient responds with "true" or "false." In order to elicit 10 responses at this level, five newspaper advertisements are included in each set.

Set A

NOTHING BEATS THE BEAN. A SUPERB BLEND,
RICH IN BRAZILIAN COFFEES. CUSTOM GROUND
8 O'CLOCK
BEAN COFFEE
3 lb bag 8.89—Save 2.40   2.99 1 lb bag

1. This is an advertisement for a soft drink. (False)
2. One pound costs less than four dollars. (True)

ASSORTED FLAVORS
FRONTENAC ICE CREAM
1/2 GALLON CTN
1.49

1. More than one ice cream flavor is available. (True)
2. The ice cream is sold in one gallon containers. (False)

GROUND FROM 100% BEEF
REGULAR GROUND BEEF
.99 per lb
Limit 10 lbs per family purchase

1. Lean beef is being advertised. (False)
2. The advertisement says that quantities are unlimited. (False)

ASSORTED FLAVORS
SEALTEST ASSORTED POPSICLES
pkg of 24   1.99

1. There is a limit of two packages per customer. (False)
2. The popsicles come in packages of 24. (True)

(single 24 oz. btl   .79—save .30)
PERRIER WATER
CASE OF 12
24 oz. btls   7.99

1. This is an advertisement for tonic water. (False)
2. The drink costs $8.99. (False)

Set B

PARTLY SKIMMED
2% FRESH MILK 1 quart bag
2.49
Limit 2 per family purchase

1. This is an advertisement for bagged milk. (True)
2. There is a limit to the number of bags purchased. (True)

Assorted Varieties
HOSTESS POTATO CHIPS
7 oz. bag
.89
Limit 2 per family purchase

1. This is an advertisement for rippled potato chips. (False)
2. The limit is two bags per person. (False)

Product of U.S.A.
Canada No. 1 Grade
SWEET CANTELOUPES
LARGE SIZE 18
each .99

1. Ontario cantaloupes are being advertised. (False)
2. Each canteloupe costs $.99. (True)

Frozen
CHICKEN DRUMSTICKS
Sold in 10 lb. ctn. @ $10.90
.99 per lb.

1. Various chicken pieces are being advertised. (False)
2. The chicken is fresh. (False)

Wink, Tonic Water, Club Soda, or Regular or
Sugar Free Gingerale or 'C' Plus Orange
CANADA DRY SOFT DRINKS
26 oz. Btl.
3/.99 (Plus .30 each bottle deposit)
Limit 6 per family purchase

1. These soft drinks are sold in bottles. (True)
2. More than one kind of soft drink is available. (True)

Level 2

Stimuli. Brief newspaper clips; 30 to 45 syllables in length; true/false statements

Procedure. The patient reads a short newspaper item. True/false statements about its content are provided in printed form or may be auditorily presented. The patient responds with "true" or "false." Two items are included in each set at this level in order to elicit 10 responses.

Set A

LONDON'S UNEMPLOYMENT RATE IS HIGHER THAN THE NATIONAL AVERAGE FOR THE FIRST TIME IN YEARS, RAISING CONCERNS THE CITY'S LUSTER AS A "GOOD EMPLOYMENT" CITY IS FADING.

1. London's unemployment rate is equal to the national average. (False)
2. This is only the second time in years the unemployment rate has been this high. (False)
3. The unemployment rate in London is considered to be a problem. (True)
4. London has a reputation for a low rate of unemployment. (True)
5. Ways of increasing employment are suggested. (False)

ARNE TREHOLT, A FORMER NORWEGIAN DIPLOMAT AND JUNIOR GOVERNMENT MINISTER, HAS BEEN SENTENCED TO 20 YEARS IN PRISON FOR SPYING.

1. Arne Treholt is currently a diplomat. (False)
2. Arne Treholt worked in Norway. (True)
3. Arne Treholt served as a government minister for 20 years. (False)
4. Arne Treholt now has a criminal record. (True)
5. Arne Treholt was arrested for tax evasion. (False)

Set B

TEXAN GARY KEHRER, A WORLD CHAMPION IN THE BLOWN

ALCOHOL HYDRO CLASS, WILL COMPETE IN THE MOLSON DRAG BOAT CHALLENGE THIS WEEKEND AT FANSHAWE LAKE.

1. This is an article about rowing. (False)
2. Gary Kehrer is a Texan. (True)
3. Gary Kehrer has only won local competitions. (False)
4. Gary Kehrer will be the judge at the Molson Drag Boat Challenge. (False)
5. The competition will occur on a lake. (True)

ST. PETER'S BASILICA, A LONDON LANDMARK ALMOST FROM THE DAY 105 YEARS AGO WHEN CONSTRUCTION BEGAN, IS 100 YEARS OLD.

1. This is an article about Rome. (False)
2. St. Peter's Basilica is usually overlooked by Londoners. (False)
3. St. Peter's Basilica is 100 years old. (True)
4. St. Peter's Basilica was built 105 years ago. (False)
5. It took five years to build the Basilica (True).

Level 3

Stimuli. Newspaper articles; 200 to 250 syllables in length; true/false statements

Procedure. The patient reads a newspaper article. True/false statements about its content are provided in printed form or may be auditorily presented. The patient responds with "true" or "false." One article is included in each set, followed by ten true/false statements.

Set A

MONTREAL (CP)—Pop singer Tony Bennett expects to open next week's Montreal International Jazz Festival with a repertoire that, like the singer, has stood the test of time.

"Jazz is America's classical music—and one of its building blocks is the popular song," says the 58 year old vocalist whose first professional engagement dates back to 1940.

The choice of Bennett and crooner Mel Torme to open and close Canada's premier jazz event appears odd to some, but not to the man once described as the most widely admired American popular singer since Frank Sinatra.

"Miles Davis became famous with great Sinatra songs like Time After Time and My Funny Valentine," Bennett observed in a telephone interview from an exclusive lunchtime eatery in Los Angeles.

"These are not old songs—they're timeless works of art."

1. The International Jazz Festival will take place in Montreal. (True)
2. This article states that people generally don't associate Tony Bennett with jazz. (True)
3. Tony Bennett says that jazz is better than classical music. (False)
4. Tony Bennett's career began in the 1930's. (False)
5. The Jazz Festival will be closed by Frank Sinatra. (False)
6. Tony Bennett claims that Miles Davis is as famous as Frank Sinatra. (False)
7. Frank Sinatra sang the song "Time After Time." (True)
8. The interview with Tony Bennett was conducted over the telephone. (True)
9. Tony Bennett gave this interview in Montreal. (False)
10. Mel Torme was having lunch with Tony Bennett during the interview. (False)

Set B

BELFAST (UPI)—A bomb in a van exploded Friday in downtown Belfast during lunch hour, sending shards of glass flying and injuring dozens of people. The Irish Republican Army claimed responsibility in a telephone call to the Republican Press Office. Police said the bomb exploded near a government building that was to be visited by Law and Order Minister Nicholas Scott.

Police began clearing the area after a warning was telephoned to local fire officials, but the bomb went off 10 minutes ahead of schedule, showering strollers with glass. Dozens were treated for cuts and shock but no one was seriously injured.

In Newry, south of Belfast, a police officer with the Royal Ulster Constabulary remained in serious condition Friday after he was shot in the chest Thursday outside the station. The IRA again claimed responsibility.

1. A bomb exploded in a large truck. (False)
2. This story took place in Belfast. (True)
3. The bomb exploded in a rural area. (False)
4. The Irish Republican Army denied any involvement in the accident. (False)
5. No people were killed. (True)
6. The police suspect that Nicholas Scott planted the bomb. (False)
7. People were injured by glass. (True)
8. The police were warned in advance about the bomb. (True)
9. A policeman was also injured in Newry as a result of a bomb. (False)
10. The policeman was fatally injured. (False)

Additional Levels

Additional levels may be developed by increasing the length and complexity of the material. Other variables to be altered would include vocabulary, redundancy, grammatical complexity, cohesion, anaphoric reference, and topic familiarity.

Chapter 6

Treatment for Gestural and Gestural-Verbal Communication

Some aphasic patients demonstrate severely limited oral expressive language and are unable to rely on their verbal output to communicate messages. Consequently, they need an alternate expressive system or an augmentative system to supplement what remains of their oral language. Among the possible alternate expressive modalities is graphic expression. However, since this modality is usually more impaired than oral expression, it is an unlikely candidate to serve this purpose (Schuell et al., 1964; Porch, 1967). Another possibility is the gestural modality. According to PICA results (Porch, 1967), the gestural modality in aphasic patients is less impaired than the verbal one. Aphasic patients have been reported to use gestures in their conversational interactions (Cicone, Wapner, Foldi, Zurif, and Gardner, 1979). The use of gesture and pantomime has also been reported as a successful strategy within the verbal communication patterns of some aphasic patients (Holland, 1982; Schlanger and Schlanger, 1970). Additionally, researchers have reported some success in aphasia rehabilitation by teaching patients hand signal systems, sign language, or Total Communication (Bonvillian and Friedman, 1978; Chen, 1968, 1971; Eagleson, Vaughn, and Knudson, 1970; Guilford, Schuerele, and Shirek, 1982; Kirshner and Webb, 1981; Moody, 1982; Peterson and Kirshner, 1981; Simmons and Zorthian, 1979). Some of these systems have been used as interim communication systems until the recovery of verbal language (Eagleson et al., 1970; Goldstein and Cameron, 1952).

Others have assumed primarily an augmentative role to verbal communication (Schlanger and Schlanger, 1970), whereas still others have replaced the verbal system (Chen, 1968, 1971; Kirshner and Webb, 1981; Skelly, 1979). For these reasons the use of a gestural system to augment oral language or to replace it seems a worthwhile venture for these aphasic patients who cannot rely on spoken language for communication.

THEORETICAL MODELS AND DEFINITIONS OF GESTURE

The hypothesized success of gestural training relates to how a clinician theoretically views both aphasia and its relation to gesture. Kimura (1982) contends that gesture and aphasia derive from a common underlying motor selection problem due to left cerebral hemisphere damage. If both modalities are impaired owing to a common problem, it could be hypothesized that gestural treatment, which involves selection and sequencing of motor movements, would be no more or less successful than oral language treatment. Another viewpoint espoused by Duffy and Duffy (1981) is that the gestural and language disturbances in aphasia are manifestations of a general symbolic disorder. They cite the high correlation between verbal and nonverbal test performance as evidence for their hypothesis. Therefore, difficulties in communicating information could be expected regardless of whether a representational gestural or an oral language model were used, and to the extent that a gestural training system involved symbolic content, it would be difficult for aphasic patients. A third view, outlined by Peterson and Kirshner (1981), is that gestural impairment is part of the linguistic impairment in aphasia. Evidence used to support this view is the correlation of the gestural deficit both with the overall severity of the language impairment and with its correlation with specific language deficits, particularly reading comprehension. Using this viewpoint, it would be expected that the more severe the overall language deficit, the more severe would be the gestural impairment. Therefore, gesture would be most impaired in those patients with the most severely limited oral expression, precisely those patients who might need a gestural system the most. Some view the expressive gestural deficit in aphasic patients as a manifestation of ideomotor apraxia. If gestural disturbance is due to ideomotor apraxia, the extent to which motor movements could be trained would dictate the possible benefits of a gestural system. De Renzi, Motti, and Nichelli (1980) reported that 80 percent of their aphasic patients demonstrated ideomotor apraxia and 53 percent were severely impaired.

The intent of this chapter is not to resolve the theoretical issue but rather to acquaint the clinician briefly with the differing viewpoints. To complicate matters further, the literature on gesture is fraught with confusing results due to differing definitions of gesture, different assessment techniques and tests, different testing contexts, different scoring systems, and so on. Perhaps defining the term gesture at this point would be helpful, since it has been used to encompass many types of motor behavior. Gesture that accompanies speech has been termed gesticulation if the motor behavior involved hand or body movements and termed mimicry if the movements involved facial expression. Natural expressive gestures are natural motor reactions to a situation (e.g., covering one's ears when the noise is too loud), whereas conventional gestures are conventionalized movements that are not direct action representations of the situation (e.g., saluting) (Goodglass and Kaplan, 1963). Motor behavior occurring in the absence of speech, used to communicate messages, has frequently been called pantomime.

Gestures may be static by involving a body part held in a fixed position, such as the V for victory sign, or they may be dynamic by involving hand or body movement, such as placing the fingers and thumb in a closed ring position and moving the hand from an imagined plate to the mouth and back, the Amer-Ind gesture for "eat." There is no necessary one-to-one correspondence between gesture and concept, although this is often the case—one gesture representing one concept, such as "house." A sequence of gestures may be required to represent a single concept, as in the case of the concept "bank" in Amer-Ind, which is represented by the combination of "house" and "money."

TREATMENT WITH GESTURAL SYSTEMS

Treatment using a gestural mode with aphasic patients has employed a variety of systems, extending at least as far back as the 1950s. Goldstein and Cameron (1952) described the Hand Talking Chart, which used differing hand configurations to represent 20 basic messages, such as "I'm thirsty." Eagleson and colleagues (1970), using a similar system, reported success in teaching 12 manual self-care signals to 31 expressive aphasic patients. No empirical evidence for effectiveness is offered in these articles, and the positive benefits are described only anecdotally. Chen (1968, 1971) designed a manual communication method for aphasic patients that combined his manual alphabet with gestures. Of 19 aphasic patients who were trained with his system, 7 demonstrated good results, 7 fair results, and 5 poor results. Sensory aphasic individuals, reportedly, were unable to learn the system at all.

Providing gestural and pantomime experiences for aphasic patients has also been reported to have positive therapeutic effects (Schlanger and Schlanger, 1970). Direct pantomime training for a group of aphasic subjects showed significant positive effects for pantomime reception and expression both on trained items and in generalization to untrained items compared with no training in a control group (Schlanger and Freemann, 1979).

The Amer-Ind Sign System

A more elaborate sign system, Amer-Ind, developed by Skelly (1979; Skelly, Schinsky, Smith, Donaldson, and Griffin, 1975; Skelly, Schinsky, Smith, and Fust, 1974), has been used with aphasic patients in several studies with some reported success (Rao and Horner, 1978; Simmons and Zorthian, 1979; Skelly, 1979). Some patients have benefited significantly and positively from Amer-Ind training; that is, they were able to comprehend and spontaneously produce signs to improve their communication. Some patients learned the signs but did not spontaneously initiate them for expressive communication. Other patients were not successful in learning or using Amer-Ind signs. (For a more complete discussion, see Peterson and Kirshner, 1981.) Therefore, Amer-Ind appears to be a potential system to consider as an alternate mode to verbal communication. It can be incorporated into LOT with some modifications and therefore is described more fully here. Reference to the original sources is necessary for obtaining the signs and for suggestions on how teaching has been done with several groups of patients (Skelly et al., 1974, 1975; Skelly, 1979).

Amer-Ind is a signal system or code based on the hand signals used by the Indians of North America. It is not a language because it does not have a rule or grammatical system. It can be adapted for unimanual use· and therefore can be employed with hemiplegic patients. The gestures are largely iconic and are reported to be clear to the interpreter. In this way they are purported to be easy to learn. Some of the gestures are static (e.g., bowl) and others are dynamic (e.g., eat). One gesture can represent several related items; for example, the gesture for *bowl* represents basin, container, dish, and receptacle. The specific meaning would be determined from context. The 250-plus signal dictionary (Skelly, 1979) can be supplemented by combining gestures to illustrate a concept. For example, the signals for "look" and "box" could be combined to represent "television." Because there is no syntax the aphasic patient does not need to be concerned about rules for combining elements. Series of signals can be combined to communicate more complex messages and often the order of the signals will indicate the semantic relationships of agent, object, and so forth.

Because the Amer-Ind signals must be learned, the principle of using 10 different items at the same level of difficulty for each trial in LOT does not apply. Hierarchies can and should be arranged to facilitate learning, using general learning paradigms. However, the acquisition criteria should be nearer 90 percent rather than 70 percent, and care should be taken to insure learning of all items, since this represents new learning rather than stimulation of previously learned material.

Gestural Language Systems

A few studies have used a gestural language system, ASL (Ameslan or American Sign Language), with aphasic patients. Bonvillian and Friedman (1978) reported that their aphasic subject learned 79 signs and used them appropriately. Concurrently, his social behavior improved. Kirshner and Webb (1981), combining ASL and Amer-Ind, reported their subject learned in excess of 100 signs and began to sequence them in communication. Guilford and colleagues (1982) alternated ASL and Amer-Ind in their therapeutic regimen with eight aphasic patients. Which system was used did not affect learning; the aphasic patients either learned both (N = 6) or learned neither (N = 2). Moody (1982) also reported success in using Total Communication with one aphasic patient.

Gestures have been classified using many different systems. One of the most complete systems, which remains relatively manageable from this author's viewpoint, was described by Cicone and colleagues (1979). The part of the body involved in the gesture movement was divided into limb, head, and torso and whole body components. The spatial properties of the movement involved its location in space, its direction of movement, and its location in personal space. The information-bearing value of gestures was coded into referential gestures, those that carried some information about things in the world, versus nonreferential gestures, which related to emphasis or rhythm. Referential gestures were subdivided into iconic, noniconic, and others. Iconic gestures in some way bore a relationship with the referent and included emblems (e.g., thumbs up for "yes"), pantomimes (e.g., holding the arm outstretched with the hand palm up and bending it toward the body for "come here"), numbers (e.g., showing three fingers for "3"), and writing (e.g., spelling a word in the air). Noniconic gestures pointed out referents. They were specific (e.g., pointing to an object) or general (e.g., pointing out two places to refer to the presence of two things rather than one). Other gestures were those that could not be listed in the other categories but were information-carrying.

Although Cicone and co-workers (1979) used spoken utterances to divide aphasic individuals' statements into propositional and nonpropositional categories, the same division could be applied to gestural sequences. Gestures would be considered propositional if the action and the arguments associated with that action were gestured. Nonpropositional gestures would include assents, denials, and sequences in which no action could be identified. Cases were assigned to gestures using Fillmore's case grammar (1968, 1975). The cases included were agent, dative I, dative II, essive, benefactive, instrumental, objective, locative, and temporal. Finally, the authors classified the clarity of spoken propositions. However, this could as easily be applied to gestures. Therefore, clarity was divided into clear (understood by partner) or unclear (incomplete or unclear reference, unclear construction, out of context).

Other parameters have also been used to classify gestures. Gestures have also been divided into representational, which include symbolic gestures (e.g., saluting or throwing a ball), and nonrepresentational, which include unfamiliar meaningless gestures (e.g., touching one's forehead with a thumb) (Kimura, 1982; Poizner, Bellugi, and Iraqui, 1984). Some have also dichotomized gestures into simple and complex categories. The simple category involves gestures that are punctate and involve little embedding, whereas the complex category involves frequent embedding.

Gestural tasks may involved body movements, such as saluting, or object manipulation, such as pounding with a hammer. Beukelman, Yorkston, and Waugh (1980) reported that aphasic patients' performance was better for body movements than for object manipulation, which has significant implications for treatment. The nature of the gestures chosen, whether they were symbolic or nonsymbolic, whether they involved finger or hand movement, whether they were static (holding a fixed position) or dynamic (involving a motor sequence), did not appear to be crucial factors influencing the performance of left hemisphere-damaged aphasic patients. What appeared to be crucial to the ability to perform the gesture was whether a patient had to organize a sequentially ordered motor program on command; that is, volitionally (De Renzi, Motti, and Nichelli, 1980). This position agreed with Critchley (1939), who proposed that it was the propositionality of the gesture that was the most important factor in performance.

The foregoing information points out that the topic of gestural communication is far from simple. Its myriad facets make it difficult to plan treatment and raise the issue of whether aphasic patients should be trained in gesture at all. However, the reality is that the oral expressive language of a group of aphasic patients is too limited to be serviceable alone. Gesture has shown some promise of success. Therefore, the gestural and gestural-verbal modality was designed to accommodate these individuals in treatment.

GENERAL GUIDELINES FOR GESTURAL AND GESTURAL-VERBAL COMMUNICATION

This modality focuses on communication, that is, getting the message across. It uses the concepts of "speech acts" and semantic relations expressed by aphasic patients. The gestures used by a patient receiving training in this modality may entirely replace spoken language. In this case, the aphasic individual is using gestures only to convey information, and to be successful, therefore, must employ one or more types of referential gestures. If gesture accompanies vocalization, the successful communicator will employ referential gestures and may add nonreferential (facial expression) gestures for emphasis. The nature of the vocalization can also add information about the illocutionary force. When gesture accompanies spoken language, the role of gesture may be to reinforce the concepts spoken (e.g., gesturing "drink" while saying "drink"), to cue spoken language (e.g., gesturing "drink," which in turn elicits the spoken word "drink"), or for emphasis (e.g., gesticulations accompanying spoken words). In all cases cited, the aphasic individual, despite severely limited spoken language, may be an effective communicator.

For aphasic patients who can rely on verbal language this modality of treatment is not considered. Although gesture might clarify or add emphasis to the verbal messages they produce, this group of aphasic individuals would more appropriately receive treatment outlined in the oral expression modality. For aphasic patients whose verbal output is severely restricted or nonexistent, treatment might begin with this modality, transferring to the oral expression modality when the patient has received some success with the speech acts area.

The areas in this modality are hierarchically organized according to supposed difficulty. Since the organization was necessarily based on clinical experience owing to the paucity of experimental research, it should be considered tentative. The clinician may find that a particular aphasic patient has no more difficulty with one area than with the following one. For example, one aphasic subject may be able to use complex pantomime as easily as simple speech acts. Therefore, some overlap in difficulty between adjacent areas is expected, but an aphasic person who cannot gain the attention of a listener is unlikely to be able to use simple pantomime.

More than one area may be included in treatment at a given time, but adjacent areas, such as gaining attention and acknowledgment of a listener message, would be most appropriate. The general progression is designed to be attraction of and maintenance of attention, then nonverbal expression, then combined verbal and nonverbal expression. The focus is on communicating messages rather than on their structure.

In the two previous modalities, the emphasis has been on describing the stimuli presented to the aphasic patient and in controlling stimulus variables as a means to exert control over the difficulty of a task. With the remaining modalities the focus will be on responses, because the aphasic patient will be expressing messages via gesture, spoken language, or written language.

Because many aphasic individuals are hemiplegic, the clinician may be concerned about using a gestural system when a patient has only one hand available, since limb movements comprise the great majority of naturally occurring gestures accompanying speech in both aphasic and normal control patients (Cicone et al., 1979; Duffy, Duffy, and Mercaitis, 1984). However, gesture systems frequently use only one limb or they can be adapted so that they can be used with one limb (Skelly, 1979; Poizner et al., 1984). When possible, most aphasic patients will choose their dominant hand, but hemiplegia will force many to use their nondominant hand. Although use of the nondominant hand does not affect the performance of normal subjects (Duffy and Duffy, 1981), the presence of sympathetic dyspraxia may affect the performance of some aphasic subjects.

Area 1: Attention

Responses. The aphasic patient inititates a response to secure the attention of the communication partner. It may be a response in a single modality or a combination. Gaining attention is an elementary step in the communication process. It may be gained through

Eye contact
Touch
Vocalization
Gesture, or any combination of these

Description. The aphasic subject gains the attention of a listener by some method other than the traditional one of using verbal language.

Example. The aphasic patient touches the clinician on the arm to attract attention.

Area 2: Acknowledgment of Message Received

Responses. The responses of the aphasic patient employ a single modality or a combination to indicate that a message has been received. Responses in this area do not imply that the message was comprehended. Responses are

Head nod
Head shake
Vocalization
Gesture

Description. The aphasic patient acknowledges that the listener has sent a message. The response signals that the patient did not understand the message, that the message was received, or that the listener sent the incorrect information.

Example. The aphasic patient shakes his or her head and waves a hand from side to side when the clinician indicates having four children. The aphasic person is signaling that the wrong information was sent: the clinician actually has two children.

Area 3: Gestural Communication

1. Single Gestures

Responses. Aphasic patients, like normal speakers, can communicate information with naturally occurring gestures, such as facial expression. The research work that has been carried out for facial expression suggests that aphasic patients are as expressive as their normal counterparts and that their facial expressions are as accurately perceived as those of normal individuals (Buck and Duffy, 1980; Duffy and Buck, 1979; Jenkins, Jiménez-Pabón, Shaw, and Sefer, 1975). One of the features that Buck and Duffy cite as perhaps important in this maintained capacity is that facial expression is not intentional; it occurs as a natural consequence to a situation.

Beukelman and colleagues (1980) found that body movements were more accurately performed than object manipulation tasks in response to three different types of instructions. This would suggest that aphasic patients might also initiate body movement responses more easily than manipulating objects. Many highly overlearned gestures might therefore be easier than performing an action involving the use of an object.

Propositional gestures have been reported to be more difficult than nonpropositional ones (Buck and Duffy, 1980; Critchley, 1939). Therefore, systems such as Amer-Ind that employ propositional gestures would be expected to be more difficult for aphasic patients than systems using appropriate facial expression.

The gestural responses below are hierarchically arranged.

Easy	Appropriate facial expression
↓	Conventional gestures
Difficult	Propositional gestures

Description. Responses in these activities require the aphasic individual to use a single simple gesture to communicate a message.

Example. The aphasic patient knits his or her eyebrows and frowns to indicate that he or she does not understand as the clinician is reading a paragraph. The aphasic patient holds his or her nose trying to communicate the fact that a skunk sprayed the neighborhood the previous evening.

2. Gesture Combinations

Responses. Responses in this section are combinations of gestures used to communicate more complex messages. If a small number of gestures are used, this is classified as simple pantomime. The use of structurally complex gestures and the concatenation of many gestures would compose complex pantomime. Amer-Ind gestures would also apply in this section.

Netsu and Marquardt (1984) reported that objects and action picture stimuli evoked better gestural performance than line drawings. In treatment, it would be wise to use the former in stimulus arrays.

The pantomime behavior of aphasic patients has been found to parallel their verbal behavior (Cicone et al., 1979; Duffy et al., 1984) Therefore, different pantomime profiles would be expected from Broca's and Wernicke's aphasic groups. The profiles in Table 6–1 represent the compilation of Cicone and colleagues' (1979) and Duffy and co-workers' (1984) work.

Description. These activities are more complex than simple gestures. The aphasic patient uses series of gestures to portray a sequence of events or to portray a complex single event, such as playing the piano.

Example. The aphasic subject pantomimes falling down and being taken to the hospital in an ambulance.

Area 4: Simple Speech Acts

Speech acts, first introduced in the language literature by Searle (1969), are concerned with the use of language in linguistic context (conversational context). They account for the linguistic content of the message and what the speaker's message intended. As such, speech acts are composed of a proposition (content) and an illocutionary force (how the speaker intended the message to be taken). Consequently, speech acts go beyond the linguistic structure of a sentence and indicate language use.

1. Communicating Illocutionary Force

Response. Illocutionary force can be signaled with a gesture or through vocalization. It refers to whether the aphasic individual intends to issue a command, to make a statement, or to question.

Table 6–1. Pantomime Profiles According to Type of Aphasia.*

Gesture Variable	Aphasic Type	
	Broca's	Wernicke's
Accuracy of communication with gesture	55 percent	57 percent
Amount of gesture	Sparse	Abundant
Rank order of frequency (most to least)	Limb Head Mouth Torso	Limb Head Mouth Torso
Time to produce response	17.5 sec	16.4 sec
Rate of movement	0.6/sec	3.0/sec
Type of movement	Slow to initiate; one-shot gesturing; mostly referential and iconic gestures; mostly clear	Almost continuous motion; about one half referential with a tendency toward noniconic gestures; many off-target and undifferentiated movements affecting clarity
Complexity	Simple	Complex
Effort	Effortful	Without effort
Smoothness	Fragmented	Smooth
Pausing	Frequent long pause	Few pauses; gesturing almost continuous

* Adapted from Cicone, Wapner, Foldi, Zurif, and Gardner (1979) and Duffy, Duffy, and Mercaitis (1984).

		Gesture	Intonation
Easy	Assertion	Slight forward drop to head with a return to original level position.	Even intonation contour with a drop at the end of vocalization.
	Command	Slight tilt back to head followed by a sharp drop.	Sharply rising and falling intonation contour.
	Question	Raised head and knitting of brow.	Rising intonation contour at the end of vocalization.
Difficult			

Description. These activities are designed to assist the aphasic patient to communicate the intent for a message, that is, whether making a statement, issuing a command, or asking a question. This helps the listener to narrow down the type of communication although it does not provide content. For example, a rising intonation pattern would signal the aphasic person is asking a question, but additional information is required to determine what question is being asked.

Example. The aphasic patient uses vocalization with a rising intonation contour while pointing to a picture whose name cannot be remembered. This signals asking the clinician for the name of the picture.

2. Communicating Content

Responses. To signal the content of messages in speech acts the aphasic person can use a simple pointing gesture or a series of pointing gestures. It is convenient ot use a case analysis approach (Fillmore, 1968, 1975) to code the semantic function of the message content. Cicone and associates (1979) found that the most frequent cases used by aphasic patients were (in order of decreasing frequency) the following:

Case	Description	Example
Dative II	The being, usually animate, affected by the verb in an experiential way; also, the noun in an existential construction.	I want that. There is **something** missing.
Agent	The animate active instigator of an action.	A **man** ate the cake.
Locative	The location or spatial orientation of the state or action named by the verb.	We went to **New York.** **Miami** is **south** of **Tampa.** She studies in the **library.**
Objective	Anything representable by a noun whose role in the state or action named by the verb depends on the meaning of the verb itself.	I wrote a **check.**

Semantic functions can also be combined as in the following examples:

    Agent—Action (verb)
    Action—Object
    Agent—Object

When presented with an array of possibilities to serve as responses, care should be taken with plausible distractors, that is, nontarget responses that might be plausible in the communication circumstances. Seron and coworkers (1979b) found that in interpreting gestures, aphasic subjects were likely to select the plausible distractor when they failed to choose the correct target.

Description. Through pointing gestures the aphasic patient is able to communicate single semantic functions, such as object, action, and agent, in the environment. Pointing coupled with an action gesture (or pointing to a referent depicting the action) permits communication of simple semantic relationships, such as an agent and action.

Example. An aphasic man points to pictures of a *boy* (agent) and then *wash* (action) to communicate the information that his son washed his car.

3. Communicating Illocutionary Force and Content

Responses. Responses here represent a combination of the responses in the preceding sections in this area. Therefore, the aphasic patient combines illocutionary force with the propositional content. Most often this will be the combination of a vocalized intonation contour plus a gesture for the content.

Description. Activities here represent a logical progression from the previous two sets. They are designed to have the aphasic patient communicate both components of a speech act—illocutionary force and content. The patient can now communicate the type of message being sent as well as its content.

Example. The aphasic patient uses a sharply rising and falling intonation contour plus points to the picture of a pen, indicating the desire to use one.

Area 5: Speech Acts

In this area, the aphasic patient increases the complexity of communication by combining verbal and nonverbal aspects. Although the patient cannot communicate effectively with verbal communication alone, supplementing verbal production with extraverbal behavior (intonation and/or gesture) increases communication. In some cases, the extraverbal behavior replaces speech (e.g., the patient gestures "hat" when she or he cannot name it), and in others it supplements speech (e.g., the patient gestures "hat" while saying it).

1. Single Word and Gestures

Responses. In this section, the aphasic patient combines a single word plus a gesture to communicate various semantic relationships. The relationships have been indicated in two systems for clinicians who may be more familiar with one than the other. They are not hierarchically arranged and are among the most common types of relationships that make up simple sentences.

Semantic Relationship	Case Analysis
Agent—Action	V—Agent
Action—Object	V—Objective
Agent—Object	Agent—Objective
Action—Location	V—Locative
Object—Location	Objective—Locative
Action—Instrument	V—Instrumental
Possessor—Possession	Dative I—Objective
Direct Object—Indirect Object	Objective—Dative II

The gesture used may correspond to the propostion (content of the message) or to the illocutionary force (the intent of the speaker).

Description. Activities within this section are more advanced than previous ones. They are designed to elicit a combination of gestural and verbal response to enhance communicative effectiveness. The goal is to have the aphasic patient communicate relationships between objects, events, people, and actions.

Example. The aphasic patient points to herself or himself and uses the word "fall" to indicate having a fall yesterday.

2. More Complex Combinations

Responses. The aphasic individual now combines three aspects in communication. The verbal portion is still relatively simple, with a single word or two that communicate a portion of the content of the message. The intonation pattern corresponds to the illocutionary force, that is, the intent of the speaker—making an assertion, asking a question, or issuing a directive. The gestural portion may be a single gesture or a combination of gestures. It carries the burden of the content to be communicated.

Description. Although the verbal aspect of this area is still relatively simple, the aphasic patient is now incorporating three aspects into the message: using content words combined with gestures and intonation pattern to express semantic relationships.

Example. The aphasic person uses a sharply rising and falling intonation pattern to the word "dog," while simultaneously communicating that the dog was a bad dog the previous day.

Chapter 7

Materials for Gestural and Gestural-Verbal Communication

Area 1: Attention

Beginning Levels

Level 1

Procedure. A therapy task is selected. Prior to presentation of a stimulus, the patient must make eye contact with the clinician. Ten trials are provided.

Level 2

Procedure. A therapy task is selected. Prior to presentation of the stimulus, the patient must make eye contact with the clinician. When a stimulus is being presented, an awareness of the task must be demonstrated.

Level 3

Procedure. A therapy task is selected. Prior to presentation of the stimulus, the patient must make eye contact with the clinician. When a stimulus is being presented, an awareness of the task must be demonstrated, along with any form of an attempted response.

Area 2: Acknowledgment of Message Received

Beginning Levels

Level 1

Procedure. When the patient is looking away, the clinician orally provides some information. The patient acknowledges reception of the message by looking toward the clinician.

Level 2

Procedure. The clinician orally provides some information to the patient. The patient is required to signal through a head shake or nod that the message has been received. Ten trials are provided.

Level 3

Procedure. The clinician orally provides some information to the patient. The patient is required to signal through any form of vocalization that the message has been received. Ten trials are provided.

Area 3: Gestural Communication

1. Single Gestures

Beginning Levels

Level 1

Stimuli. Pictures of situations associated with a variety of emotions or feelings

Emotion or Feeling

1. fatigue
2. fear
3. pensiveness
4. pleasure
5. dislike
6. sympathy
7. surprise
8. anger
9. pain
10. unhappiness

Procedure. The clinician presents a picture associated with a particular emotion or feeling. An appropriate facial expression is provided by the clinician to be imitated by the patient. The series of pictures is then reviewed, with the patient required to provide the facial expression without a model.

Level 2

Stimuli. Pictures depicting situations associated with conventional gestures

Gesture

1. licking lips: tastes good
2. rubs stomach: hungry
3. holding arms: cold
4. fanning face: hot
5. waving: extending a greeting
6. finger to lips: be quiet
7. pinching nose: unpleasant smell
8. thumbs down: bad
9. hands over ears: noisy
10. circle made with thumb and index finger: "okay"

Procedure. The clinician presents a picture depicting a situation associated with a conventional gesture. The gesture is provided by the clinician to be imitated by the patient. The series of pictures is then reviewed, with the patient required to provide the gesture without a model. Gestures may be modified for execution with one hand, in the case of hemiplegic patients.

Level 3

Stimuli. Pictures depicting actions associated with propositional gestures

Actions

1. eating
2. drinking
3. washing
4. driving
5. cooking
6. combing hair
7. writing
8. sleeping
9. coming
10. running

Procedure. The clinician presents a picture depicting an action associated with a propositional gesture. The gesture is provided by the clinician to be imitated by the patient. The series of pictures is then reviewed, with the patient required to provide the gesture without a model.

Single Gestures: Additional Levels

Additional levels might be developed by eliminating the pictured stimuli and designing communication situations in which the patient is required to provide information to the clinician through a single simple gesture. A hierarchy can again be developed from facial expression through conventional gestures to propositional gestures.

2. Gesture Combinations

Beginning Levels

Level 1

Procedure. Action pictures are presented, with the patient required to execute two gestures associated with information in the picture.

Level 2

Procedure. Short newspaper articles are presented to the patient. The patient is required to communicate the main ideas through a series of gestures. If reading comprehension problems preclude performance of this task, videotape segments depicting various situations could be used.

Level 3

Procedure. The clinician asks the patient questions requiring factual information to be communicated through a series of gestures. Topics both familiar and meaningful to the patient are selected: for example, "What did you do in your garden this morning?"

Gesture Combinations: Additional Levels

Additional levels may be developed by increasing the demand placed on the patient to communicate through gesture; that is, requiring the patient to communicate through gesture at times other than during task presentation.

Area 4: Simple Speech Acts

Beginning Levels

Level 1

Stimuli. Action pictures

Procedure. Through pointing gestures, the patient is required to communicate one of the following semantic functions contained in the picture:

agent-action, action-object, or agent-object. The patient must point to the agent and object in the picture or point to the agent-object and demonstrate the action. Ten presentations are provided.

Level 2

Stimuli. Pictured objects or actions

Procedure. The clinician presents a pictured item to elicit assertions, commands, and questions. The patient is required to name the picture, using an even intonation contour, with a drop at the end of vocalization. If unable to name the item, vocalization, with a rising intonation contour, is required. To signal readiness for the next stimulus presentation, a sharply rising and falling intonation contour must be used. Opportunities are provided to elicit 10 assertions, commands, and questions.

Level 3

Stimuli. Action pictures

Procedure. The clinician presents an action picture to elicit assertions, questions, and commands. The patient signals assertions through pointing to items in the picture while vocalizing with an even intonation contour, with a drop at the end of vocalization. The clinician then asks for information not appropriate to the content of the picture. While pointing to the picture, the patient vocalizes, using a rising intonation contour at the end of vocalization. The patient signals readiness for the next stimulus presentation by pointing to a new picture, while vocalizing using a sharply rising and falling intonation contour. Opportunities are provided to elicit 10 assertions, commands, and questions.

Area 5: Speech Acts

Beginning Levels

Level 1

Stimuli. Action pictures

Procedure. The clinician presents an action picture. The patient is required to communicate information about some aspect of the picture by providing at least one word in combination with an appropriate gesture. For example, for a picture of a boy eating, the patient might say "boy" and gesture "eating."

Level 2

Stimuli. Action pictures

Procedure. The clinician presents an action picture. The patient is required to communicate some aspect of the picture by providing at least one word in combination with an appropriate gesture.

Level 3

Stimuli. Action pictures

Procedure. The clinician presents an action picture. The patient is required to communicate some aspect of the picture by providing one or more words in combination with one or more appropriate gestures. The amount of either verbalizing or gesturing must be increased at this level.

Additional Levels

Once the patient has completed this hierarchy and oral speech is increasing, the focus in treatment might shift to activities in oral expression.

Chapter 8

Treatment for Oral Expression

Aphasic patients are certainly distinguished from normal speakers by their oral expressive language. In fact, characteristics of oral expression exclusively were used to classify aphasic patients earlier in our history (Benson, 1967). Oral expressive language characteristics remain important today as major contributors, along with auditory comprehension, in a variety of classification systems for aphasia.

The types of deficits in oral expression vary among aphasic patients, as does the severity of deficits. A moderate Broca's aphasic patient will sound quite different from a moderate Wernicke's patient. However, they will share many common areas of difficulty, such as word retrieval problems, phonological articulatory deficits, and so on.

The areas of deficit, their severity and nature, are important parameters of treatment planning. As with other modalities, oral expression was divided into several mutually exclusive areas. The first area involved language production at a highly overlearned or automatic level (Automatic Speech Series). The second concerned the phonological-articulatory aspects of verbal production (Phonological-Articulatory Production), and the third was Repetition. What these three areas share is that they do not require the active formulation of propositional utterances. Oral reading and oral spelling, Areas 4 and 5, although not frequently used skills by most people in their verbal production, can serve as alternate or supplementary routes for the aphasic patient to accomplish reading and writing tasks. The last four areas (Naming, Area 6; Oral Formulation, Area 7; Conversation, Area 8; and Discourse, Area 9) compose the majority of oral expression tasks, since they deal with semantic and syntactic processing of meaningful language. Explanatory material for all areas has been provided as background information for the clinician, with the exception of Area 1, Automatic Speech Series, which appeared self-explanatory.

PHONOLOGICAL-ARTICULATORY PRODUCTION

Listening to the spontaneous speech or verbal production during test per formance of many aphasic patients reveals the frequent presence of misarticulations. These articulation errors may be the result of phonological, articulatory, or a combination of phonological-articulatory problems. The terms apraxia of speech and verbal dyspraxia are frequent labels for these problems seen in patients with anterior left-hemisphere lesions in and surrounding Broca's area. Although phonological-articulatory problems are seen in isolation, they are most often accompanied by aphasia and are viewed by some as being part of the syndrome of Broca's aphasia (Blumstein, Cooper, Goodglass, Statlender, and Gottlieb, 1980; Canter, 1969; Shewan, 1980a, 1980b; Shewan, Leeper, and Booth, 1984; Trost and Canter, 1974). These problems also are manifested as articulation errors in patients with posterior left-hemisphere lesions. Frequently referred to as phonemic or literal paraphasias, they are typically found in conduction and Wernicke's aphasic patients, although to a lesser degree in the latter group (Burns and Canter, 1977; Goodglass and Kaplan, 1972).

In conjunction with Broca's aphasia, researchers are in general agreement about the symptoms presented, although the underlying causes are still debated. One group believes that the articulation errors are the result of programming problems in the sequencing of the neuromotor commands that drive the articulatory musculature (Darley, 1970; Darley, Aronson, and Brown, 1975; among others). Another group believes that the phonological component of the linguistic system is also involved, thereby resulting in phonological as well as phonetic errors (Blumstein, Cooper, Zurif, and Caramazza, 1977, 1980; Itoh, Sasanuma, and Ushijima, 1979; Monoi, Fukusako, Itoh, and Sasanuma, 1983; Shewan, 1980a; Shewan et al., 1984). The symptoms most frequently described are consistent phonemic substitutions, phonetic errors, groping for correct articulatory postures, particular problems with place of articulation, and increasing difficulty across vowels, single consonants, consonant clusters, and longer stimuli.

Traditionally, the phonological-articulatory errors of posterior lesion patients are described as phoneme selection problems, which result in inconsistent phonemic substitutions in speech (Canter, 1969). These errors occur in the context of fluent speech with conduction aphasic patients, who are usually aware of their errors (Kohn, 1984), and Wernicke's patients, who are frequently unaware of their substitutions. Recent investigations have supplied some evidence that conduction and Wernicke's problems may not be limited only to phonological errors but also may include phonetic errors as well (Blumstein et al., 1980; Shewan et al., 1984).

Whether the problems are the result of motor programming difficulties or are of linguistic origin has theoretical implications for the nature of aphasia and presumably for the treatment of these disorders. MacKenzie (1982) recommended differential treatment patterns for the two groups of patients. Unfortunately, there are no data available regarding whether the auditory discrimination approach that she recommends for fluent patients is successful. For the present, speech-language pathologists seem to be at the stage where symptoms are treated rather than the underlying processes, and further research is necessary to refine treatment programs.

REPETITION

Repetition activities are standardly included in aphasia test batteries. Performance on repetition tasks provides useful diagnostic information about type of aphasia. The transcortical aphasias (transcortical sensory, transcortical motor, isolation) are characterized by their comparatively superior repetition performance, whereas conduction aphasia is characterized by inferior repetition performance.

In treatment, repetition tasks are included in some treatment programs, but not in all. The patient's repetition of stimuli is not usually the end goal of treatment; rather repetition serves as a transition to spontaneous speech. Repetition activities may be beneficial in facilitating performance in other aspects of oral expression. In severely dyspraxic patients, who produce only stereotyped utterances, it forms the first stages of Multiple Input Phoneme Therapy (Stevens and Glaser, 1983). It has been successfully used in the beginning stages of treatment for verbal dyspraxic problems in patients with greater verbal output (Shewan, 1980b). Treatment that included repetition and word retrieval components had a positive impact on both these aspects of oral expression in a case study, whereas treatment of word retrieval alone did not (Sanders, Davis, and Hubler, 1979).

Repetition forms an integral part of Melodic Intonation Therapy (MIT) that was introduced to speech-language pathologists by Albert, Sparks, and Helm (1973). This method was based on the observation that some aphasic patients maintained the ability to sing but were severely non-fluent for oral expressive language. The authors hypothesized that combining speech with intonation patterns would facilitate regaining oral expressive language. The method stresses intoning patterns of propositional phrases or sentences, which resemble one of the several natural, logical possibilities for English. It controls the elements of stress, melodic line, and rhythm in the patterns. Intoned patterns are slower than normal speech rate, with a precise rhythm and distinct stress. As aphasic patients progress through the program they assume more independence from the clinician by delaying repetition of the clinician's intoned pattern and transitionalizing to the spontaneous production of patterns. The units also become longer and there is a gradual transition from melodic intonation to normal speech prosody.

MIT is not advocated with all aphasic individuals. Reported to be the best candidates are aphasic patients with good auditory comprehension relative to their verbal expression, who possess self-monitoring skills, have difficulty with repetition, but continue to attempt to communicate. These characteristics appear consistent with a description of verbal dyspraxia.

The method has been outlined in detail in several articles to which the reader is referred for more complete information about how to use MIT (Sparks, 1981; Sparks, Helm, and Albert, 1974; Sparks and Holland, 1976). A large scale efficacy study remains to be reported for MIT. Sparks and associates (1974) reported that 6 of 8 patients who received MIT regained some appropriate propositional language. The patients served as their own controls, since they had made no improvement in verbal expression with traditional language therapy for at least six months prior to instituting MIT. Sparks (1981) reported that studies extending MIT results to include about 45 aphasic patients ". . . make it possible to predict that about 75 percent of carefully selected candidates will realize the predicted degree of language recovery" (p. 266).

The use of MIT might be considered for appropriate aphasic patients who do not respond to the areas of LOT outlined below. MIT could be used as a branch program with resumption of LOT in the area of oral formulation when MIT has been completed.

ORAL READING AND SPELLING

In Chapter 4, several forms of dyslexia were mentioned. Although dyslexia refers to reading difficulties, several forms are characterized by certain symptoms present in oral reading. Therefore, a brief review of these varieties of dyslexia (or alexia) will orient the clinician to diagnosing them and consequently to providing appropriate treatment.

Coltheart's classification (1982) refers to four types of dyslexia: pure alexia, phonological dyslexia, surface dyslexia, and deep dyslexia. These types are identified by using a stimulus-response paradigm in which the most potent stimulus variable and the aphasic patient's response are identified.

Pure Alexia

The pure alexic patient is characterized by having difficulty with reading increasingly longer words. She or he appears to adopt a letter-by-letter reading approach as a method to achieve meaning. Spelling and writing are intact, and this type of alexia has also been referred to as alexia without agraphia and posterior alexia. Letter naming is usually somewhat defective although letter identification may be intact. Aphasia may be absent although color agnosia and right homonymous hemianopsia often accompany pure alexia.

Surface Dyslexia

This type of dyslexia is characterized by poor spelling of irregular words. Because the semantic route to reading is damaged, the patient has to rely on the orthographic-phonological route. Although this route may be effective for regular words and nonwords, it cannot handle irregularly spelled words. These patients tend to make regularization errors in their reading and to spell phonetically. Therefore, "gnome" might be spelled "nome," "board" might be "bord," and "yacht" might be "yot."

Phonological Dyslexia

Patients with phonological dyslexia have the most difficulty with reading nonwords. They must be spelled and read by applying orthographic-phonemic correspondence rules, since they are not represented in the semantic lexicon. Because this route is damaged they cannot read nonwords. They make many visual errors in reading, confusing letter strings that look similar, but they do not make semantic errors.

Deep Dyslexia

These patients are characterized by several symptoms: (1) They make semantic errors in reading aloud (e.g., chicken/egg, woman/girl); (2) they read content words more accurately than functor words (e.g., dog versus on); (3) they read concrete words better than abstract ones (e.g., house versus hope); and (4) they cannot read nonwords (e.g., ganterless). In addition to semantic errors, a necessary condition for this type of alexia, these patients make visual errors and derivational errors (e.g., wisdom/wise, direction/directing). Some researchers have also reported visual-then-semantic errors in which the word read appears to be semantically related to a word visually similar to the target (e.g., sympathy/orchestra, presumably via symphony). This type of dyslexia is always accompanied by aphasia, usually Broca's, and usually associated with right hemiplegia. Word reading is usually superior to letter reading (e.g., "bee" but not b).

ANOMIA

Another aspect to the oral expression deficit is that of anomia, or word-retrieval problems. Difficulty in recalling the name of an object occurs in all types of aphasic patients, although anomia also occurs in nonaphasic disorders. Everyone is all too familiar with anomia, as when caught in the embarrassing situation of being unable to recall an acquaintance's name during an introduction.

For many years aphasiologists recognized word finding problems in patients but there was little attempt to subdivide them further. Today it is clear that not all word-retrieval problems reflect the same impairment, and it is important to recognize different types, as treatment will differ. Although there are other classifications of anomias (Geschwind, 1967; Luria, 1966), Benson (1979) has detailed five varieties associated with aphasia and four that are nonaphasic in nature. To provide background for the naming section later in this chapter each will be outlined briefly.

Word Production Anomia

Motor

Patients with this type of anomia know the word (name) they want to produce, but they cannot produce it or they produce it incorrectly. These patients cannot initiate the motor patterns necessary to produce the word, and this word-finding difficulty is often accompanied by articulatory problems and groping for the correct articulatory targets. The patient can frequently produce the word when cued with the initial phoneme and may be able to write the word. Because the word seems to be available at some level, whether these problems should be viewed as word-retrieval problems is debatable. Patients with these problems often demonstrate Broca's aphasia. This anomia may also be mixed with word selection anomia described further on.

Paraphasic

Another type of word production anomia is characterized by words containing phonemic paraphasias. Depending on the number of paraphasias in each production, the target word may or may not be recognizable. Frequently, this type of anomia mimics the "tip-of-the-tongue" phenomenon, because the aphasic can recognize the word immediately when provided by the examiner and often has some knowledge about the word, its first letter, number of syllables, and/or correct intonation pattern (Goodglass, Kaplan, Weintraub, and Ackerman, 1976).

Word Selection Anomia

Benson also referred to this as word dictionary anomia. The patient knows the meaning of the word and can describe the object or its function but cannot produce the name or may produce it inadvertently and not realize it. The patient immediately recognizes the word when provided and can select the word when given a choice. These patients often fail to respond to cueing. This type of anomia is frequently accompanied by fluent, circumlocutory, empty speech.

Semantic Anomia

These patients cannot retrieve the word and also fail to understand the name when it is provided (spoken or written). They often fail to respond to or echo the examiner rather than name the word. Their expressive language is fluent and empty and auditory comprehension is poor.

Category-Specific Anomia

Although rare and rarely occurring in a pure form, anomia in these patients is limited to words of a particular category. Most frequently reported is color anomia (Geschwind and Fusillo, 1966), although other categories can be involved (Yamadori and Albert, 1973).

Modality-Specific Anomia

Patients with this type of anomia fail to name objects presented in a particular modality, most often the visual modality, although tactile and auditory modalities could also be involved. As with word production anomias, there is some question about whether these should be referred to as word-retrieval problems, although symptomatically they manifest themselves as such.

Nonaphasic Anomias

Anomias due to disconnection result from lesions separating the hemispheres (corpus callosum) or intrahemispheric disconnections. The word-retrieval problems of dementia, especially Alzheimer's disease, are differentiated from aphasic anomias by their initial selective impairment of naming as tested in word fluency tasks (divergent naming) and later impairment in confrontation naming tasks (convergent naming). Nonaphasic misnaming often associated with acute confusional states is usually transient. The misnamed words are often illness related and may appear confabulatory (e.g., waiter/doctor; hotel/hospital). Psychogenic anomia is very rare and usually accompanied by otherwise normal speech. Patients may misname common objects yet produce a complex description of their occupations using technical and rare vocabulary.

ORAL FORMULATION

Oral formulation involves the production of meaningful grammatical units, usually sentences. Aphasic patients frequently have difficulty with sentence formulation and the problem is particularly prominent in Broca's and Wernicke's types.

Broca's subjects are often described as demonstrating telegraphic speech because they have a heavy loading of content words with fewer functor words when compared with normal adults. They do not totally ignore functor words but they do not appear to understand their syntactic functions, with the result that functors are often misplaced in sentences. Broca's aphasic patients also produce short simple sentences on the average, with little variation in grammatical form and with morphological errors. Their prosody is abnormal, with a loss of normal intonation pattern. They speak at a slow rate, overall output is reduced, and their speech is frequently described as effortful and labored. As recovery takes place, their sentences become more complex and there is a increase in the number of grammatical markings per sentence (Myerson and Goodglass, 1972).

Wernicke's aphasic patients distinguish themselves by their fluent, copious output, which frequently lacks content (and therefore is often called empty) or contains many paraphasias, which may interfere with conveying a meaningful message. Their sentences are normal in length and they express a variety of grammatical forms. Prosody and speech rate are normal, with the noticeable lack of struggle that is characteristic of Broca's patients. They violate grammatical rules at all levels, making their expressive language difficult to understand. Wernicke's patients are frequently unaware of their errors and their failure to communicate with their conversational partner.

Global aphasic patients produce little output, usually single words and perhaps a stereotyped utterance (e.g., "oh dear"). They frequently make no response to requests requiring expressive language output.

Anomic aphasic patients maintain the syntactic aspects of production. Prosodic and length features are normal, as is the variety of grammatical forms available. Because they have significant word-retrieval problems their speech may be characterized by general terms (e.g., thing, this, do, make) where more specific referents are required. This has been referred to as empty speech. Their verbal output may also be circumlocutory or contain many revisions as they struggle with word-finding difficulties. However, they are usually able to communicate their message.

Conduction aphasic patients also are described as fluent. They have most difficulty in achieving the correct phonemic form of words. Consequently, their speech contains many phonemic paraphasias. They are aware of their difficulties and often try to correct them, resulting in reapproaches to the word (conduite d'approche). Their sentence length, variety of grammatical forms, and speech rate are within normal limits. They may sound hesitant owing to the large number of reapproaches to the correct target production.

CONVERSATION AND DISCOURSE

The last two areas in oral expression are termed Conversation and Discourse (originally Extended Narrative). Although both represent different forms of discourse, or connected language, they were separated into two categories for several reasons: (1) to differentiate between the presence and absence of a conversational partner, (2) to recognize differences in the communicative acts expressed, and (3) to acknowledge the give-and-take exchange of dialogue versus monologue. When LOT was formulated, there were no data about the differences in aphasic patients' performance with various types of discourse. This has been included here to provide the clinician with an up-to-date view of this aspect of oral expression.

By way of introduction, *discourse* is a term that has been used in a general sense to refer to connected language. Some authors have divided discourse in to several categories such as conversation, narrative, procedure, and expository. Each category has its own set of operating rules, called a discourse grammar. Of course, sentential grammar (a set of rules describing sentence form) applies to all types of discourse.

The structure of conversation can be described using more than one system. Gurland, Chwat, and Gerber-Wollner (1982) used Geller and Wollner's communication profile, which divided conversation into conversational acts and communicative acts. Conversational acts functioned to initiate, extend, and terminate interactions or topics. Communicative acts conveyed content (requests, comments, instructions, responses, performatives), regulated conversation (organizational devices), and expressed attitudes. Turn-taking and maintenance of topic or topic shifts are also important aspects of conversational exchanges. Holland and co-workers (1982) used the Systematic Analysis of Language Transcripts (SALT) system to analyze conversation. Although the measures concentrated on quantitative aspects of verbal production, such as the total number of complete utterances, the groups of conversational facilitators, tanglers, and metaconversational features focused more on language use measures.

Narrative discourse refers to the description of a happening, expressed using a sequence of events or episodes. An episode has a distinct structure with essential and optional components. The outline below (from Ulatowska, North, and Macaluso-Haynes, 1981) follows the conventional order although variations occur.

1. *Abstract*. This refers to a description of what the narrative is about. It is optional.
2. *Setting*. This describes the time, location, and background of the episode and identifies the participants. It is essential.
3. *Complicating Action*. This describes the events that take place. It is essential.
4. *Evaluation*. This refers to an evaluation of the events. It is usually included but not essential.
5. *Resolution*. This refers to what finally happened or the outcome. It is essential.
6. *Coda*. This refers to the moral of the story. It is essential.

Procedural discourse refers to connected language whose purpose is to describe a procedure or the steps involved in how to do something. Procedural discourse is goal-oriented, with the set of steps chronologically or conceptually linked (Ulatowska, Doyel, Stern, and Macaluso-Haynes, 1983a).

1. Introduction (Optional)
   This refers to describing what the procedure is about.
2. Steps (Essential)
   a. Essential steps are those actions necessary to accomplish and understand the task.
   b. The target step shows that the procedure is complete.
   c. Optional steps
      i. Auxiliary
         At the same level as essential steps, these extend beyond the essential.

ii. Substeps
These are subordinate to essential steps and add detail.
3. Evaluation (Optional)
This is less common than in the narrative.
4. Resolution (Optional)
5. Coda (Optional)

Expository discourse is primarily subject-matter oriented. It does not have a personal reference or a chronological order although the topics are logically related and cohesion is maintained.

Discourse can also be analyzed using a sentential grammar approach, which evaluates the quantity and quality of verbal output. Semantic and syntactic measures are also applicable here. Quantity is generally measured by the total number of words and/or utterances produced, length by the mean length of utterance or clause, and complexity by measures of embedding and complexity of sentence structure.

Semantic aspects of discourse are as important as structural ones. Ulatowska and colleagues (1981) used measures of content and clarity to approach this aspect of discourse. Their content rating represented a rough equivalence to coherence. Coherence is a general cognitive concept that relates to the plausibility, conventionality, and cohesiveness of the discourse. Their clarity rating was a rough measure of cohesion. Cohesion refers to the use of various linguistic devices, such as anaphora and reference, to link items in discourse together.

The use of conversation and discourse areas in treatment is important, as these areas more closely represent the type of language used in daily settings, that is, functional language.

Area 1: Automatic Speech Series

Responses. When aphasic patients demonstrate extremely limited verbal output and are unable to generate oral language spontaneously, the latter may be facilitated by using automatic or highly overlearned speech. Aphasic patients may differ in their production proficiency for the following categories; however, no data are available to support a hierarchical arrangement:

Greetings
Counting
Poems
Days of the week
Months of the year
Alphabet

A variant of automatic speech production has been described by Helm and Barresi (1980) in which an aphasic patient's involuntary stereotyped utterances are brought under voluntary control and their production progresses from automatic involuntary production to conversational speech.

Description. Activities in this area are designed to elicit highly automatic or serial speech. They would be used as an attempt to facilitate verbal output from aphasic patients who produce little or no voluntary speech. It is hoped that these activities proceed to the use of more functional language.

Example. The aphasic patient uses greetings appropriately upon arriving to the clinic or when meeting clinic personnel.

Area 2: Phonological-Articulatory Production

Many variables are important to control in phonological-articulatory treatment programs. Shewan's (1980b) content network (Table 8–1) for a verbal dyspraxia treatment program served as the basis for LOT training in this area. It was based on the work of many authors and has been supplemented with additional research data (Blumstein et al., 1977; Burns and Canter, 1977; Dunlop and Marquardt, 1977; Goodglass, Fodor, and Schulhoff, 1967; Green, 1969; Hardison, Marquardt, and Peterson, 1977; Johns and Darley, 1970; Kearns, 1980; MacKenzie, 1982; Martin, 1973; Martin and Rigrodsky, 1974a, 1974b; Mercaitis and Duffy, 1984; Monoi et al., 1983; Rosenbek, Lemme, Ahern, Harris, and Wertz, 1973; Shankweiler and Harris, 1966; Shewan, 1980a; Tonkovich and Marquardt, 1977; Trost, 1970; Trost and Canter, 1974).

Stimuli. The stimuli for production or repetition have been studied by many researchers. As the content network hierarchy shows, the phonemic content, length, frequency of occurrence, and linguistic factors affect accuracy of production. When productions are not accurate, substitutions are the most frequent error type. Distortions do occur in both groups, although they are less frequent in the fluent group (MacKenzie, 1982; Shewan et al., 1984). For most aphasic patients, consonants occasion more errors than vowels, although Monoi and colleagues (1983) reported an equal number of vowel and consonant errors for a group of conduction aphasic patients. Metathetic errors are most frequent in the fluent patients (Monoi et al., 1983), whereas transitionalizing errors are most common in the Broca's group (Trost, 1970; Trost and Canter, 1974).

At the single consonant and syllable levels, highly frequent phonemes result in fewer errors than less frequent phonemes. Within consonants, there is a hierarchy of difficulty for Broca's and fluent groups as indicated,

Table 8-1. Content Network for Verbal Dyspraxia Treatment Program*

Stimulus Presentation Method	Stimuli	Responses	Facilitating Response Variables	Criterion Response

A. Auditory
  Auditory model
  Phonetic placement
	Hierarchy from Easy to Difficult
	A. Vowels, diphthongs
		A. Clinician-initiated
		  Number
		    Single response
		    Multiple responses
		  Time
		    Unison
		    Immediate repetition
		    Delayed repetition
		  Propositionality
		    Automatic
		    Drill context
		    Responsive
		      Responsive to question
		      Sentence completion
		    Spontaneous
			A. Slow speech rate
			B. Altered prosody
			C. Compensatory movements
			  Approximations
			D. Associated Responses
			  Body movement
			  Tapping
			  Rhythmical activity
				A. Qualitative
				  Correct
				  Intelligible
				B. Quantitative
				  70% or more correct over
				  2 blocks of 10 items each

B. Visual
  Watch clinician
  Mirror use
    Provides visual
    feedback to client
  Graphic presentation
  Written words
  Anatomical charts
	B. Single consonants
	  Hierarchy from easy to difficult
	    Nasals m, n
	    Glides l, r
	    Plosives p, t, k
	    Fricatives, affricates
	    h, s, z, t, tʃ, ʃ, dʒ
	    Dentals θ, v
	  Distinctive features			

C. Tactile Motokinesthetic Method	Hierarchy from easy to difficult
	  Nasality
	  Voicing
	  Manner
	  Place
		B. Client-initiated
		  Spontaneous
		    Length
		    Complexity
		    Phonologic
		    Syntactic		

D. Multimodal
  Auditory-visual
  Auditory-tactile
  Visual-tactile
  Auditory-visual-tactile
	C. CV, VC combinations
	  C + Different V
	  Different C + V
	  Vary C and V			

	D. CVC monosyllabic words
	  Variables to control
	    Frequency of occurrence
	    Concreteness
	    Meaningfulness
	    Length
	    Functionality			

	E. Single words with C clusters			

	F. Bisyllabic words, two word combinations
	  Both syllables or words with primary stress
	  Initial word or syllable only with primary stress
	  Final word or syllable with primary stress			

	G. Syntactic units
	  Length
	  Linguistic complexity
	  Phrases
	  Sentences
	  Active
	  Passive			

*Adapted from C. M. Shewan (1980), Verbal dyspraxia and its treatment, **Human Communication, 5,** 3–12.

although not found in the fluent group by MacKenzie (1982). Using distinctive feature analysis, errors for Broca's aphasic patients are generally only one distinctive feature removed from the target, although they are either one or two distinctive features removed for fluent aphasic patients. A difficulty hierarchy for distinctive features shows that nasality and voicing tend to be maintained to a greater extent than manner and place. Fricatives and affricates are frequently produced as stops, whereas palatal and dental consonants occasion more errors than consonants with other places of articulation.

At the single word levels (C, D, E, and F of Table 8–1) several additional variables are important to control. Functional words produce fewer errors than nonfunctional ones. Concrete words are produced more accurately than abstract ones, and high frequency words are produced more accurately than low frequency words. Length of the stimuli is also important. In general, more errors occur as the stimulus length increases either in the number of phonemes or syllables, although the increases are not linear. That real words produce fewer errors than nonsense words stresses the importance of introducing meaningful material as soon as possible. The position of errors in single words has produced conflicting results. For Broca's aphasic patients, some studies have indicated more errors in the initial position, whereas others have not found any differences across initial, medial, and final positions. In fluent aphasics, Burns and Canter (1977) and MacKenzie (1982) found most difficulty with the final position.

With linguistic units beyond the single word level, length, stress, and linguistic complexity are important variables to control. Frequency of occurrence will continue to exert an effect on the words within the longer unit. Primary stress facilitates accurate production, as does short length. At the sentence level, active sentences are more accurately produced than passives, and more errors occur on the first noun phrase (NP$_1$) than the second noun phrase (NP$_2$) in sentences.

A variety of presentation methods have been outlined in the content network. They are not presented in hierarchical order although it has been demonstrated that auditory-visual presentation results in more accurate productions than with either modality presented alone. Comparison of auditory and visual (picture, written word) presentation revealed equal error rates. The rule of thumb is to provide as much stimulus support as is necessary for the patient to achieve some success and to gradually reduce stimulus support when it is no longer needed. Auditory presentation includes providing an auditory model for the patient or providing verbal instructions with regard to phonetic placement. Visual presentation may involve a visual model provided by the clinician or anatomical charts, self-monitoring using a mirror, or presentation of the written word. Tactile presentation involves the clinician providing tactile placement cues or actually manipulating the patient's articulators as in what has been called the motokinesthetic method in articulation therapy.

Responses. Responses can be divided into clinician-initiated and client-initiated, with the latter being more difficult. Within clinician-initiated responses, the number of responses requested, whether a single response or multiple responses following the stimulus, and the timing of the stimulus and response, from unison to immediate repetition to delayed repetition, scale responses from easy to difficult. As propositionality of the response increases from an automatic drill context to spontaneous production, the difficulty for the patient increases. Client-initiated responses are more difficult for patients because no model is provided and they are generally highly propositional. Both length and complexity of the responses are important variables to control to achieve success.

Facilitating response variables are responses used in addition to speech or speech alterations to facilitate accurate response productions. As the patient becomes able to produce responses without these facilitators, they can be eliminated. If required and effective, they can continue to be used by the patient. Reducing speech rate has been effective with some patients, thereby increasing intelligibility. Although a slow speech rate may alter prosody, with a tendency to equalize stress, this may result in a more intelligible response than using a faster speech rate. Prosody may be normalized at a later stage in treatment as the patient is able to accommodate it. Some phonemes and consonant clusters may be produced with compensatory movements; inserting a schwa between consonants in a cluster is a common example. Accurate motor production may be facilitated by accompanying speech with associated movements, such as finger tapping.

The notion of criterion response is familiar by now. It refers to the setting by the clinician of criteria for what will be an acceptable response. Qualitatively, this may refer to correct or intelligible responses, and for LOT, achievement of 70 percent or more correct responses over two blocks of 10 items each defines the quantitative criterion for progressing to the next level of difficulty in the hierarchy.

Description. The goal for activities in this area is to improve the aphasic patient's phonological-articulatory productions. By using the content network, illustrated in Table 8–1, and advancing in a step-by-step fashion, the patient approaches the spontaneous production of propositional speech. The support from the clinician is gradually reduced as the patient achieves established performance criteria, thereby demonstrating the ability to function more independently. The patient proceeds as far as possible through the hierarchy. For some, this may fall short of normal speech production.

Example. The aphasic patient has difficulty producing labiodental phonemes. The clinician stresses correct placement for /f, v/ in the context /__a/ and gradually increases the difficulty of the phonetic context to other syllables, words, and so on.

Area 3: Repetition

Stimuli. The stimuli to be repeated have an effect on the responses produced by aphasic patients. Several linguistic factors have been reported to influence repetition accuracy. As length of the items increases, performance declines (Gardner and Winner, 1978); the inverse relationship has been found for probability. High probability sentences are generally repeated more accurately than low probability ones (Goodglass and Kaplan, 1972, 1983). Meaningful items are more easily repeated than nonmeaningful ones or nonsense words (Davis, Foldi, Gardner, and Zurif, 1978; Martin, Kornberg, Hoffnung, and Gerstman, 1978).

Both type of items and type of aphasia influenced repetition performance, although auditory comprehension did not (Gardner and Winner, 1978). Anterior lesion patients performed more poorly than posterior lesion ones and also made more sound errors in repetition. By contrast, conduction aphasic subjects made a high number of meaning errors and responded differentially to the types of items listed. The hierarchy (Gardner and Winner, 1978) lists those items easiest to repeat first and the types of aphasia from most accurate production performance to least accurate.

		Example
Easy	One-digit numbers	six
	Nouns	car
	Grammatical words	a, beside, and
	Two-digit numbers	forty-two
	Letters	s, w
	Fractions	¾
	CV monosyllables	/ba/
	Three-digit numbers	one hundred thirty-four
	Percentages	sixty-two percent
	Nonsense words	/hɔrta/
Difficult	Money	three dollars and fifty-five cents

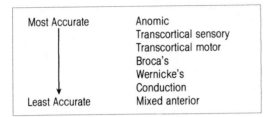

Most Accurate	Anomic
↓	Transcortical sensory
	Transcortical motor
	Broca's
	Wernicke's
	Conduction
Least Accurate	Mixed anterior

The semantic and syntactic composition of sentences affects repetition in transcortical aphasic patients. Davis and co-workers (1978) reported the following rank ordering of sentence types from most to least accurate repetition.

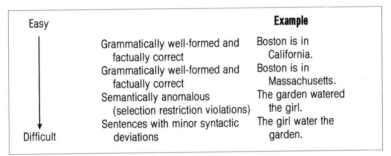

Easy		**Example**
↓	Grammatically well-formed and factually correct	Boston is in California.
	Grammatically well-formed and factually correct	Boston is in Massachusetts.
	Semantically anomalous (selection restriction violations)	The garden watered the girl.
Difficult	Sentences with minor syntactic deviations	The girl water the garden.

Aphasic patients generally have more difficulty with sentences as they increase in syntactic complexity. They attempt to retain the meaning rather than retain the exact syntactic form. Goodglass's (1968, 1976) work outlines a hierarchy for various sentence forms from easy to difficult.

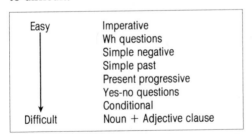

Easy	Imperative
↓	Wh questions
	Simple negative
	Simple past
	Present progressive
	Yes-no questions
	Conditional
Difficult	Noun + Adjective clause

Responses. Additional response variables important for repetition are context and the immediacy of the response. When inflected single words were included in syntactic contexts, fewer omission errors occurred compared with repetition in isolation (Martin et al., 1978). Gardner and Winner (1978) found that Broca's aphasic patients performed better when repetition was delayed for 3 seconds following presentation, whereas anomic patients performed better in the immediate condition. Other types of aphasic patients performed almost identically in the two conditions.

Martin and colleagues (1978) reported that substitution errors were the most frequent, followed by omission errors, with addition errors being least frequent. Errors also tended to be more frequent in the second consonant cluster of inflected single words in isolation, but position did not affect the same words in context. Their hierarchy is reproduced below.

Easy	Errors	Target /slæps/
↓	Substitution	/slæpt/
	Omission	/slæp/
Difficult	Addition	/slæpst/

1. Single Items

Responses
Phonemes
Letters
Numbers
Words

Description. The aphasic patient is asked to repeat the stimulus after the clinician. Activities are designed to emphasize accurate reproduction of a model provided by the clinician. The hierarchies provided are used to select appropriate stimuli.

Example. The aphasic patient is asked to repeat a number presented by the clinician.

2. Unrelated Items in a Series

Responses
Phonemes
Letters
Numbers
Words

Description. The aphasic patient must retain a series of unrelated items and repeat them after the clinician. These tasks involve accurate production while increasing memory load.

Example. The clinician auditorily presents a series of three words, and the aphasic patient repeats the three-word series.

3. Meaningful Linguistic Units

Responses
Phrases
Sentences

Description. Activities involve the repetition of meaningful linguistic units, such as phrases and sentences. Again the aphasic patient is to accurately repeat the model of the clinician.

Example. The aphasic patient repeats functional phrases used in a card game, following presentation by the clinician.

Area 4: Oral Reading

For most persons, oral reading is not a frequent activity. Therefore, its use in aphasia treatment might be questioned. Improvement in oral reading per se is generally not the goal of the treatment; rather, it is used as a vehicle to improve other language performances as discussed in this area.

Stimuli. Many variables affect the oral reading performance of aphasic patients. Because different sets of variables affect different types of the dyslexias, it is important to identify the nature of the reading disturbance.

For patients demonstrating the symptom complex of deep dyslexia, some syntactic categories are easier than others and content words are easier than function words (Coltheart, 1982; Friedman and Perlman, 1982; Kapur and Perl, 1978; Marshall and Newcombe, 1973, 1966; Sartori, Bruno, Serena, and Bardin, 1984; Shallice and Coughlan, 1980; Shallice and Warrington, 1975). High imageability words produce more accurate performance than low imageability words (Coltheart, 1982; Richardson, 1975; Sartori et al., 1984; Shallice and Warrington, 1975). Imageability refers to the extent to which an item elicits a mental image. Concreteness refers to the extent to which the referent can be experienced by the senses, and its influence on oral reading has been inconsistent. In some studies it has not been well defined and people have reported better performances for concrete words compared with abstract words. However, when imageability, word frequency, and lexical complexity (simple versus derived nouns) were controlled, Richardson (1975) found no significant concreteness effect. Context facilitates performance in at least some deep dyslexic patients (Coltheart, 1982).

Common, frequent words are read orally with greater accuracy than low frequency words (Shallice and Warrington, 1975). Nonwords are produced with greatly reduced accuracy, if at all (Friedman and Perlman, 1982; Marshall and Newcombe, 1973; Sartori et al., 1984).

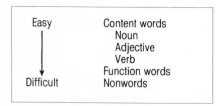

Those patients who demonstrate pure alexia (alexia without agraphia) are most sensitive to word length. As the number of letters in the word increases, their performance declines both in accuracy and latency (Benson, Brown, and Tomlinson, 1971; Coltheart, 1982; Gardner and Zurif, 1975).

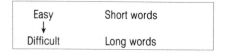

Aphasic patients demonstrating surface dyslexia have difficulty reading irregularly spelled words, that is, those not spelled phonetically (Bub, Cancelliere, and Kertesz, 1982; Coltheart, 1982; Marshall and Newcombe, 1978). They can read regularly spelled words and nonsense words well, as they read using grapheme-phoneme correspondence rules.

Easy → Difficult
Regular words
Nonsense words
Irregular words

Patients with phonological dyslexia share many symptoms with deep dyslexic patients. They can read real words but not nonwords. Whether the words are regularly spelled or not has no significant effect on performance (Coltheart, 1982). Several variables—brevity, operativity, and grammatical form class—were examined in four groups of aphasic patients. The hierarchy was similar across groups, although some differences occurred. To capture these, the hierarchy from most accurate oral reading to least accurate will be listed for each aphasic type (Gardner and Zurif, 1975).

Easy	**Broca's**	**Wernicke's**
↓	Short picturable nouns	Short picturable nouns
	Operative nouns	Operative nouns
	Figurative nouns	Short non-nouns
	Grammatical particles	Grammatical particles
	Short non-nouns	Abstract nouns
	Long non-nouns	Figurative nouns
Difficult	Abstract nouns	Long non-nouns
Easy	**Global**	**Alexia with Agraphia**
↓	Short picturable nouns	Short picturable nouns
	Grammatical particles	Operative nouns
	Operative nouns	Figurative nouns
	Figurative nouns	Short non-nouns
	Short non-nouns	Grammatical particles
	Long non-nouns	Abstract nouns
Difficult	Abstract nouns	Long non-nouns

As length of material increases, aphasic patients generally make more total errors in oral reading. This is understandable and predictable, simply on the basis of the greater opportunity to err in longer passages. Whether the error rate per syllable would increase has not been reported. The hierarchy for stimulus length given here is listed primarily to assist the clinician in selecting material at an appropriate level of difficulty rather than for length to be used as the primary variable to be manipulated.

Words
Phrases
Sentences
Paragraphs

Description. Activities are designed to improve the aphasic patient's ability to produce orally a corresponding written message. Various levels of difficulty have been included. The patient might be trained in this area if oral reading elicited better comprehension of written language than silent reading. Oral reading could also be used as a vehicle to improve the prosodic aspects of oral production. Passages could be marked for stress, intonation, and juncture to practice these suprasegmental aspects of phonology. Broca's aphasic patients frequently demonstrate impairment in these production aspects, giving their speech a monotonous, arrhythmic quality.

Example. The aphasic patient reads aloud a sentence that corresponds to a picture being shown by the clinician.

Area 5: Oral Spelling

As with oral reading, oral spelling is impaired to a greater degree in some patients than in others. Benson (1977) reported that his frontal and central alexia groups were impaired in this task, whereas for his posterior alexia group, oral spelling was intact. Similar findings have been reported by Coltheart (1982) for pure alexia with retained oral spelling and for deep dyslexia with impaired oral spelling (Goldberg and Benjamins, 1982; Shallice and Warrington, 1975).

Stimuli. Aphasia test batteries generally include a series of words for oral spelling. These range fron short, highly frequent, phonetically spelled words to longer, less frequent, irregularly spelled words. These are three variables to control in treatment although detailed information is not available concerning the degree of their relative impact on oral spelling performance.

Reponses. Responses can be of two types, one in which the patient completes the spelling of a word, given one or more of the letters by the clinician. The other response type entails spelling the entire word as shown:

Word Completion
Spell Entire Word

Description. Activities here require the aphasic person to spell orally words of varying degrees of difficulty. Tasks are included as an approach to aid spelling ability. Some aphasic patients find oral spelling easier than written. Also some patients, particularly those who demonstrate pure alexia, use oral spelling as a method to associate the printed word with its meaning.

Example. The clinician auditorily presents a word to the aphasic patient who spells the word orally.

Area 6: Word Retrieval or Anomia

Treatment for naming or word-retrieval problems first necessitates determining what type of anomia or anomias appear to be present. Because performance can differ depending on the task, whether describing a picture, naming to confrontation, or talking in conversation (Kreindler, Fradis, and Mihailescu, 1983; Williams, 1983), it is important to assess naming in more than one context and to account for this in treatment.

Responses. Williams (1983), in a review article on naming in aphasia, cited four major variables that appeared to influence naming performance in aphasia. Her variable list will serve as a framework here.

Characteristics of the Referent to Be Named

Gardner (1973, 1974b) reported that aphasics' naming was superior for operative items, that is, items that were manipulable, discrete, and available to several senses (e.g., book) than for figurative items, which were not manipulable, continuous with their environment, and available to fewer senses (e.g., cloud). This variable does not appear to be independent of others, such as word frequency and concreteness, which also influence word retrieval. More abstract stimuli are less easily named than concrete ones.

What semantic category an item belongs to has also been shown to affect naming (Goodglass et al., 1966). The hierarchy lists items from easiest to most difficult to name, although the differences among categories are not always statistically significant.

	Semantic Category		
Easy	**Broca's**	**Wernicke's**	**Anomic**
↓	Objects	Letters	Letters
	Actions	Actions	Numbers
	Colors	Numbers	Actions
	Letters	Objects	Colors
Difficult	Numbers	Colors	Objects

	Grammatical Category	
Easy	**Broca's**	**Wernicke's**
↓	Nouns	Verbs
Difficult	Verbs	Nouns

Mills, Knox, Juola, and Salmon (1979) reported that greater stimulus uncertainty negatively influenced naming performance response times. The more consistently an item was named using the same word by normal subjects the lower its uncertainty value. Aphasic patients took significantly longer to name high uncertainty items than low uncertainty ones. Whether frequency of occurrence confounded results could not be determined, since this variable was not controlled.

Another semantically related variable is prototypicality, or how characteristic an item is of its class. For example, an apple is very prototypical for the category fruit, while a tomato is much less so. During divergent naming tasks (word fluency) Grossman (1978) reported that Wernicke's mean prototypicality scores were higher than for Broca's aphasic individuals. Although both groups started naming with high prototypical members, Wernicke's subjects went further and further afield, occasion-

ally going out of the category, while Broca's patients followed low prototypical items with high ones. Asked to name prototypical and nonprototypical line drawings of *cup, bowl,* and *glass,* Broca's subjects were
sensitive to prototypicality, the name applied coinciding with perceptual
features characteristic of each label. Less consensus in naming was
achieved in boundary zones in which the drawings were nonprototypical.
Anomic aphasic subjects, however, did not respond to prototypicality
(Whitehouse et al., 1978).

Whether semantic complexity and markedness would affect naming
performance was examined by Drummond, Gallagher, and Mills (1981).
Using two production tasks of sentence completion and antonym production, which were equivalent in difficulty, subjects produced adjectives that
varied in semantic features and markedness. Of a pair of polar opposite
adjectives, the one that is more complex is termed marked, whereas the one
that is less complex is termed unmarked. The unmarked adjective of the
pair refers to both a point on the dimension and the entire scale of values
(e.g., long), whereas the marked member (e.g., short) refers only to a point
on the dimension. Aphasic subjects produced a significantly greater number of unmarked adjectives in the sentence completion task, with no differences evident for the antonym production task. The semantic feature
hierarchy for the two tasks based on the mean percentage of correct responses is shown below.

Easy	**Antonym Production**	**Sentence Completion**
	Age (animate)	Speed
	Goodness	Age (inanimate)
	Happiness	Age (animate)
	Speed	Height
	Height	Goodness
	Length (inanimate)	Length (inanimate)
	Distance	Happiness
	Length (animate)	Distance
	Age (inanimate)	Size
	Size	Width
	Width	Depth
Difficult	Depth	Length (animate)

Characteristics of the Referent's Name

Various parameters of the name of the referent influence aphasic
patients' naming performances. Frequency of occurrence has been well
documented in this regard. Corlew and Nation (1975) found it to be the
single best predictor of naming ability in a study examining 21 stimulus
variables. High frequency words are named more accurately than low frequency ones (Corlew, 1975; Gardner, 1973; Li and Canter, 1983; Oldfield

and Wingfield, 1965; Rochford and Williams, 1965; Wepman, Bock, Jones, and Van Pelt, 1956; Wingfield, 1968).

Length of the name affects both accuracy and latency of response. As length is increased by adding letters, syllables, or both, performance of aphasic patients becomes slower and less accurate (Barton, 1971; Gainotti, Micheli, Silveri, and Villa, 1983; Goodglass et al., 1976; Venus, 1975, cited in Williams, 1983).

Pronounceability of the referent name, as determined by ratings of normal subjects, affected fluent aphasic subjects' accuracy and latency of response; however, no effect was seen for nonfluent aphasic subjects (Corlew, 1975). Since pronounceability is highly correlated with word frequency (Spreen and Schulz, 1966), it is difficult to separate the effects in Corlew's data. Stressed words are more likely to be included in a recall task by Broca's aphasic patients than are nonstressed words. They seem to use a strategy of searching for a stressed word to initiate utterances (Goodglass, 1976).

Type of Stimulus Presentation

The stimuli that are used to elicit the naming responses can affect performance of aphasic subjects. Goodglass, Barton, and Kaplan (1986) and Goodglass (1980) reported naming difficulties for all sensory modalities of presentation—visual, auditory, tactile, and olfactory. However, as reported earlier, there are rare cases of modality specific anomias.

When visual materials are used for presentation their particular characteristics may influence naming performance, although results have not been consistent. Bisiach (1966) reported a difference with better naming to realistic representations than to line drawings, but no difference between them and drawings mutilated with crosshatching. Benton, Smith, and Lang (1972) reported significantly better naming for real objects than for small line drawings; however, this finding was not substantiated by Corlew and Nation (1975) and Hatfield, Howard, Barber, Jones, and Morton (1977). Further, Benton and co-workers found no differences between large and small line drawings, nor did Faber and Aten (1979) find any differences between pictured objects presented intact and presented in broken or altered state (e.g., a pair of glasses with a broken lens). Therefore, the following hierarchy is considered as tentative and may be pertinent only to a portion of the aphasic population.

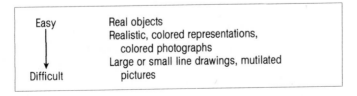

The exposure time of the stimuli to be named and the intertrial interval influenced naming performance (Brookshire, 1971). The optimal exposure time appeared to be 5 seconds, as further increases did not positively influence performance. Intertrial interval had less effect.

Context in Which Naming Occurs

The variable of context is not a unitary one, since context can refer to several aspects of naming. Stimulus context is perhaps the most frequently investigated in aphasia and interacts with other variables. When the item to be named occurs as part of a sentence completion task, this frequently results in better naming performance than confrontation naming (Barton, Maruszewski, and Urrea, 1969; Podraza and Darley, 1977; Wyke and Holgate, 1973). When the sentence can be completed by a single noun, naming was better than when the context was less specific, that is, when more than one word could complete it (Pierce, 1981). Results have not been as promising for grammatical categories other than nouns—adjectives and prepositions (Drummond et al., 1981; Friederici, 1981). Naming to description is often more difficult than confrontation naming, especially for Broca's and Wernicke's aphasia patients although not for anomic aphasic individuals (Goodglass and Stuss, 1979). When the item to be named is viewed in the context of a picture, naming is generally facilitated for some types of aphasic patients (Whitehouse et al., 1978; Williams and Canter, 1982). However, Hatfield and associates (1977) did not find a facilitating effect of context.

The difficulty context also influences naming performance. Whether an item is named corrrectly is influenced by whether the preceding items were named correctly. Brookshire (1972) and similarly Gardiner and Brookshire (1972) found that difficult items, as determined in a pretest, were named correctly when placed after easy-to-name items. Conversely, pretest easy items were more difficult when preceded by difficult items. The following are hierarchies summarizing context results. As previously, easy items are listed first.

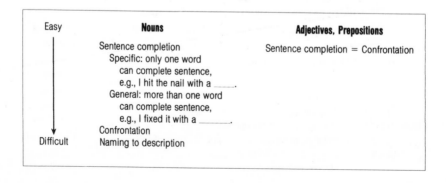

Easy	Broca's	Wernicke's	Anomic	Conduction
↓	Confrontation	Picture description	Confrontation	Picture description
Difficult	Picture description	Confrontation	Picture description	Confrontation

Because responses are not always totally correct or totally incorrect and because certain types of responses are more characteristic of certain groups of aphasia than others, the following response hierarchy is suggested. The associated responses in the semantically related paraphasia category were taken from Goodglass (1980).

Correct
1. Totally correct
2. Recognizable with phonemic paraphasia(s)
Incorrect
1. Semantically related paraphasia
    Superordinate
        e.g., clothing/sock
    Attribute
        e.g., smelly/sock
    Contrast coordinate
        e.g., shoe/sock
    Context
        e.g., baseball/sock
    Functional associate
        e.g., darn/sock
    Clang
        e.g., talk/sock
2. Circumlocutory response
    e.g., you put it on your foot/sock
3. Semantically unrelated paraphasia
    e.g., book/sock
4. Neologism
    e.g., stupick/sock
5. Indicates inability to respond
    e.g., I can't/sock
6. No response

The goal of word-retrieval activities in treatment is to improve the patient's performance and to teach ways to circumvent the problem when it occurs. Teaching the patient to use cues or strategies is a major aspect of naming treatment. The idea is to determine which cues are most effective for the patient and to have the patient gradually assume responsibility for cueing (see Chapter 1 for more detail).

Type of aphasia and severity of the naming deficit influence the effectiveness of cues (Li and Canter, 1981); Weidner and Jinks, 1983). Broca's aphasic subjects profited to a significantly greater extent from phonemic cues that did Wernicke's aphasic subjects, with conduction and anomic aphasic groups performing in between. Aphasic patients with mild naming deficits benefited more from cues than did severely impaired patients.

The following hierarchy of cues and their description is an amalgamation of information from several sources (Drummond and Rentschler, 1981; Helmick and Wipplinger, 1975; Love and Webb, 1977; Marshall, 1976; Pease and Goodglass, 1978; Podraza and Darley, 1977; Rochford and Williams, 1962). Gestural cues have been reported to assist in naming, especially when accompanied by other cues (Drummond and Rentschler, 1981; Hoodin and Thompson, 1983); however, fewer data were available, making it difficult to insert them in the verbal cue hierarchy.

Most Effective	Cue	Description
	Repetition	The target word is presented as a model for the subject.
	Delay	The subject delays before responding with a name.
	Phonemic	The initial phoneme or syllable is provided by the clinician.
	Sentence completion	A sentence is presented by the examiner with a blank for the subject to complete with the target word. The fewer the number of possible words that can complete the sentence the more efficient the cueing.
	Semantic association	A word that is semantically associated with the target word is presented by the clinician.
	Printed word	The printed target word is presented.
	Description	A description of the item is provided by the clinician.
	Rhyming word	A word that rhymes with the target is presented by the clinician.
	Situational context	A situation in which the item would be found is provided.
	Spelled word	The target word is spelled orally for the subject.
	Functional description	The function of the target item is given by the clinician.
Least Effective	Superordinate	A superordinate term is provided by the clinician.
	Generalization	A general statement that provides little specific information is given by the clinician.

Some additional features of cueing provide useful information for planning treatment. The first cue, regardless of type, was found to be the most effective (Drummond and Rentschler, 1981) when naming response time was measured. Providing multiple cues before requesting a response was more effective than the same single cues provided sequentially (Weidner and Jinks, 1983). Seron, Deloche, Bastard, Chassin, and Hermand (1979) emphasized the importance of focusing treatment on the recovery of access strategies to the lexicon to achieve generalization to untrained items, and presumably to different contexts.

Description. The goal of word retrieval is not to train responses, that is, to teach the patient new words, but rather to facilitate the processes involved in word-retrieval. Therefore, the focus is determining what cues or strategies help the client, increasing awareness of effective cues, and increasing their use.

Scoring. Double scoring for word-retrieval activities is required. First, the number or percentage of words achieving the established response criterion is scored. When this level exceeds approximately 50 percent, the clinician should increase the difficulty of the stimuli to precipitate word-retrieval problems. Since the goal is to teach cues and strategies, it is important for the aphasic patient to have sufficient opportunity to use a cueing system. The 50 percent level was selected so the task would not be overly difficult while permitting ample opportunities to use cues. Second, the effectiveness of cues in naming performance is also scored. This might include the percentage of time a cue was effective in eliciting the correct target, the percentage of time the aphasic patient initiated a cue when it was required, and so forth.

Example. (1) The aphasic patient uses phonemic cueing to name pictured items in a confrontation naming task. (2) The aphasic patient uses effective cues (previously determined in treatment) in a conversation with the clinician.

Area 7: Oral Formulation

Training in this area is designed to improve the aphasic patient's ability to generate meaningful units at the phrase and sentence level. Because some patients tend to rely on a single grammatical form, the goal can include increasing the variety of forms as well. It is important to note that the studies whose data are reported here have not always used all types and severities of aphasia. Therefore, it is important for the clinician to test each patient to determine if a hierarchy needs to be altered.

Stimuli. As with many other tasks in oral expression, the stimulus variables used can affect patient performance. Comparing a picture description task with conversational speech, Easterbrook, Brown, and Perera (1982) reported that a small group of aphasic patients used significantly more major utterances (containing a subject-predicate structure as defined by the LARSP system) with pictures as stimuli.

Presentation of picture stimuli and written words composing a sentence was compared with auditory and visual presentation of the verb (e.g., *is eating*) only in a sentence formulation task. Both methods resulted in significantly increased proportions of correct linguistic constituents (noun phrase, verb phrase, prepositional phrase) and appropriate lexical items (Shewan, 1976b).

The context in which stimuli are presented also affects the responses produced. Researchers have used contexts of sentence completion (Story Completion Test by Gleason, Goodglass, Green, Ackerman, and Hyde, 1975) and spontaneous formulation. In general, the hierarchies for these contexts are similar.

The following hierarchy from easiest to most difficult is taken from Goodglass, Gleason, Bernholtz, and Hyde (1972) and Zatorski and Lesser (1981). Since Zatorski and Lesser studied only questions and to-complements, the latter construction was placed at the end of the list. It also matches the order recommended by Helm-Estabrooks (1981) in the Helm Elicited Language Program for Syntax Stimulation (HELPSS).

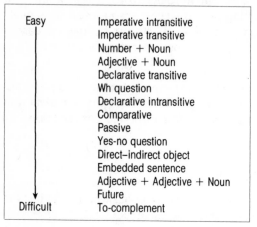

Easy

Imperative intransitive
Imperative transitive
Number + Noun
Adjective + Noun
Declarative transitive
Wh question
Declarative intransitive
Comparative
Passive
Yes-no question
Direct–indirect object
Embedded sentence
Adjective + Adjective + Noun
Future

Difficult   To-complement

It is important to note that this hierarchy is suggested as being one that is followed by many aphasic patients. However, it is important to verify this hierarchy or to establish another based on each patient's performance. This need and the importance of defining a criterion response have also been pointed out by Salvatore, Trunzo, Holtzapple, and Graham (1983).

Wales and Kinsella (1981) had Broca's aphasic patients complete sentence frames with various word classes. Although degree of contraint, whether the sentence could be completed by only one or more than one word, did not affect performance, there were differences between grammatical categories. Not all differences were statistically significant; however, the following list is rank ordered from easiest to most difficult.

Easy	Class	Example
↓	Particle nonadjacent	She switched the light **off**.
	Noun	She hit the nail with a **hammer**.
	Particle adjacent	She switched **off** the light.
	Verb	She **fed** the young puppy.
Difficult	Preposition	She goes **to** school every day.

Responses. Responses in oral formulation activities vary in syntactic complexity, length, prosody, and morphological markers included.

Aphasic patients produce sentences more accurately if they keep them short. Broca's aphasic patients are frequently limited by short phrase length. Wernicke's aphasic patients tend to make more errors in sentence predicates. Therefore, reducing length will reduce errors and increase the probability of retention of train of thought.

Agrammatic aphasic subjects have difficulty using the appropriate word order to reflect certain semantic relations (Saffran, Schwartz, and Marin, 1980) between agents and objects. The order of least to most difficult is

Easy	Agent-Object	Example
↓	Aninate-Inanimate	The boy pushes the wagon.
	Inanimate-Inanimate	The ball hit the car.
	Animate-Animate	The boy pushes the girl.
Difficult	Inanimate-Animate	The ball hit the boy.

Noted here was the difference in difficulty for sentences of different types using a sentence completion paradigm. Ludlow (1973) examined the order of reappearance of various sentence constructions during spontaneous language recovery in a group of aphasic patients. She found that the order of reappearance was highly correlated with the frequency of occurrence of the structures in normal adult language samples and that the hierarchies were similiar for Broca's and fluent aphasic patients. The order of reappearance was similar to the hierarchy of difficulty reported by Goodglass and co-workers (1972). Given this similarity, one can conjecture that the longer list of forms for reappearance can also be used as a difficulty hierarchy. It can, therefore, be used as a basis for selecting the sentence types appropriate for different levels of training. Sentence types in braces reflect reappearance at the same time.

Easy	**Example**	**Broca's**	**Fluent**
	I can't do it.	Negative placement	Negative placement
	I do not play baseball.	Do support	Do support
	He is tall.	"be" verb	"be" verb
	The cat ate the mouse.	"past" verb	"past" verb
	He said that he would come home.	Complement in VP	Complement in VP
	He hid behind the door.	Simple prepositional phrase	Simple adverb phrase
	She studies in the library.	Simple adverb phrase	Adjective modifier
	He wanted to go to the bank.	Equi. NP deletion	Progressive verb
	What is the trouble?	Wh question	Relative clause in VP
	The big car is more expensive.	Adjective modification	
	My shoe is too tight.	Possessive article	Simple prepositional phrase
			Equi. NP deletion
	He is eating a banana.	Progressive verb	Wh question
	What will he bring?	Subject-verb inversion	Adverb preposing
	Come here.	Imperative	Complement in prepositional phrase
	Every day he brings the mail.	Adverb preposing	Possessive article
			Preposition deletion
	I saw the girl who bought the car.	Relative clause in VP	Subject-verb inversion
	The dress of the lady is very sheer.	Possessive formation	Perfect verb
	I have caught the ball.	Perfect verb	Yes-no question
	I have an apple and an orange.	NP conjunction	Sentence conjunction
	The woman walks in daytime and she drives at night.	Sentence conjunction	Sentence conjunction reduction
	There is a picnic here today.	There insertion	Passive
	The lady's dress is very sheer.	Possessive shift	Reflexive
	The woman walks in daytime and drives at night.	Sentence conjunction reduction	There insertion
	I am waiting for him to return from the army.	Complement in prepositional phrase	Agent deletion
	I don't know what to do with a cookbook.	Wh complement	"It" replacement
	The apple was eaten by you.	Passive	Wh-complement
	I am afraid that he will be late.	Preposition deletion	Relative clause in prepositional phrase
	The apple was eaten.	Agent deletion	Relative clause in adverbial phrase
	I talked to the girl who bought the car.	Relative clause in prepositional phrase	Preposed NP complement
			Possessive form
	The cat washed herself.	Reflexive	Yes-no complement
	I will tell you when she returns.	Relative clause in adverbial phrase	Sentence in VP
			Particle movement
	That he came home surprises me.	Complement in NP	Possessive shift
	It is very important for him to be here.	Extraposition to VP	Complement in NP
	They will come on time, I hope.	Preposed NP complement	Relative clause in NP
	Is it hot today?	Yes-no question	Complement in adverbial phrase
	I don't know if I can come today.	Yes-no complement	Imperative
	I **do** make a good cake.	Emphatic placement	Emphatic placement
	John is certain to find out.	"It" replacement	Extraposition to VP
	He said, "I'll show you the way."	Sentence in VP	Dative
	She will come after doing the dishes.	Complement in adverbial phrase	Possessive pronoun
	That shoe of mine is too tight.	Possessive pronoun	Extraposition from NP
	She turned off the light.	Particle movement	Tag formation
	The train that goes to Y is always late.	Relative clause in NP	
	The man gave a ball to the girl.	Dative	
	That is the answer, isn't it?	Tag formation	
Difficult	The train is leaving now that stops in Baltimore.	Extraposition from NP	

Morphological markers do not appear to be of equal difficulty for aphasic patients. Using a sentence completion format Goodglass and Berko (1960) reported similar hierarchies for fluent and nonfluent patients, except that the latter made more errors and had greater difficulty with nonsyllabic endings.

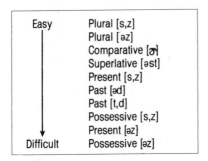

Easy — Plural [s,z]
Plural [əz]
Comparative [ɚ]
Superlative [əst]
Present [s,z]
Past [əd]
Past [t,d]
Possessive [s,z]
Present [əz]
Difficult — Possessive [əz]

A frequency of use hierarchy including different markers was reported by de Villiers (1974) for eight inflections used by nonfluent aphasic patients.

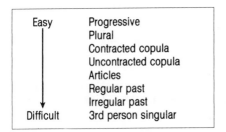

Easy — Progressive
Plural
Contracted copula
Uncontracted copula
Articles
Regular past
Irregular past
Difficult — 3rd person singular

Prosody, particularly stress pattern, influences the productions of Broca's aphasic patients (Goodglass, 1976; Goodglass et al., 1967). They frequently omit initial unstressed functor words, whereas medial functor words are much more resistant to omission. They seem to adopt a strategy of searching for a stressed word to initiate sentences.

Description. Activities in this area are designed to improve the aphasic patient's formulation of grammatical constructions rather than single word responses. The preceding variables discussed and the hierarchies presented allow the clinician to plan materials of appropriate difficulty.

Example. The aphasic patient is asked to formulate a simple active affirmative declarative sentence to correspond to a picture presented by the clinician.

Area 8: Conversation

Because conversation involves exchange, the aphasic patient both initiates utterances and responds to the utterances of others. For practical purposes, all utterances by the patient will be grouped under the response category.

Little research data are available concerning the variables that influence aphasic persons' conversation. The conversational style of the patient is important both with respect to an analysis of output and with respect to shaping the behavior of the communication partner (Gurland et al., 1982). Although Gurland and co-workers studied only two patients, both patients produced a variety of communicative acts: requests, comments, responses, and so on. Examining narrative discourse, Linebaugh, Kryzer, Oden, and Myers (1982) termed their topics as conversation because the examiner, a familiar listener, interacted with the patient during verbalization. They reported a strong positive correlation between the percentage of exchanges initiated by the patient and the overall level of functional communication as measured by the Communicative Abilities in Daily Living (CADL) (Holland, 1980). That these patients were rated as sharing more of the communication burden implied they were better communication partners. However, premorbid communication style was not taken into account.

Piehler and Holland (1984) reported different and changing cohesion patterns in the conversations of two acute aphasic patients during their early recovery.

Responses. Conversational responses consist of a variety of utterances that vary in length, complexity, communicative intent, and semantic content.

The following materials are aspects that can be evaluated in conversation. They are subjectively rank ordered for difficulty on the basis of clinical experience, but there are no corroborating research data as yet.

Length
Short utterances
Long utterances

Complexity
Phrases
Simple sentences
Complex sentences
(See previous section for hierarchy)

Topic
Familiar topic
Less familiar topic

Conversational Partners(s)
One familiar partner
One unfamiliar partner
More than one familiar partner
More than one unfamiliar partner

Setting
Familiar
Unfamiliar

Communicative Intent
Difficulty can be increased by expanding the variety of intents expressed. It is not yet clear whether some are more difficult than others because conversational style confounds the issue.

	Example
Requests	What time is it?
Comments	I bought the red car.
Instructions	Push the button.
Responses	Yes, I think so too.
Performatives	That's mine.
Organizational devices	It's my turn.
Expressives	I feel sick.

Description. Activities in this area are designed to aid the aphasic patient in producing appropriate utterances in a conversational setting. They also require the patient to keep in mind material that has occurred previously, so that responses follow the trend of the conversation.

Example. The clinician and the aphasic patient exchange information about the patient's recent vacation. The conversation might take the form of

Examiner: Where did you go?
Aphasic: To the South.
Examiner: Whereabouts in the South?
Aphasic: Florida.
Examiner: What did you do in Florida?
Aphasic: We went to the beach.

Area 9: Discourse

The majority of the work on discourse in aphasic patients, centered around narrative and procedural discourse, has been carried out by Ulatowska and her colleagues (Bond, Ulatowska, Macaluso-Haynes, and May 1983; Ulatowska et al., 1981; Ulatowska, Freedman-Stern, Doyel, Macaluso-Haynes, and North, 1983b; Ulatowska, Macaluso-Haynes, and North, 1980). They have reported that the structure of discourse was maintained in mild and moderately impaired aphasic patients although it was disrupted in severe aphasic subjects. The amount and complexity of language was reduced at all severity levels.

Stimuli. The stimulus conditions, whether highly structured as in a picture sequence or lowly structured as in an array of dolls, affected the quantity of language and level of discourse produced by aphasic patients (Lemme, Hedberg, and Bottenberg, 1984). Quantity of language increased with increasingly structured stimuli as did developmental level of the narrative, assigned using Applebee's system. The increasing developmental levels were (1) heaps, (2) sequences, (3) primitive narrative, (4) unfocused chain, (5) focused chain, and (6) narrative. However, stimulus context did not affect the syntactic level or the use of cohesion in the narratives produced by the aphasic patients.

| Easy ↓ | Low structured stimuli |
| Difficult | High structured stimuli |

The task performed influenced phonation rate and the mean duration of pauses in aphasic patients (Deloche, Jean-Louis, and Seron, 1979). Values for these variables were higher in a picture description task with a visual stimulus present than in a narrative task talking to an interviewer.

Responses. The utterances produced during narrative and procedural discourse can be analyzed using discourse and sentential approaches as described earlier. Features for mild, moderate, and severe aphasic patients shown here come from Ulatowska's work referred to previously (1983a, 1983b).

Mild	Moderate	Severe
All essential structural elements included	All essential structural elements included	All essential structural elements included
Followed chronology of events	Followed chronology of events	Failure to follow chronology of events
Participants systematically marked	Participants systematically marked	Participants unsystematically marked
Unsuccessful with morals	Considerable impairment with morals	
Reduced evaluation	Reduced evaluation	
Properly used cohesive devices	Frequent cohesion errors, primarily anaphora	

Content and clarity were also measured by Ulatowska and her colleagues. These measures were taken as estimations of coherence and cohesion.

Mild	Moderate	Severe
Reduced content	Reduced content	Reduced content
Reduced clarity	Reduced clarity	Markedly reduced clarity

Both Broca's and Wernicke's subjects showed a reduced mean number of target lexemes (content words produced by at least 90 percent of normal speakers) in the Gleason and co-workers' study (1980) as well as a reduced number of themes. A frequent cohesive error for the aphasic subjects was the production of pronouns without antecedent nouns (anaphora), making it difficult to identify the participants consistently.

Sentential grammatical analysis revealed the following information (Ulatowska and colleagues).

Mild	Moderate	Severe
Reduced quantity of language	Reduced quantity of language	Reduced quantity for anterior patients, not for one posterior patient
No. clauses	No. clauses	
No. words per T-unit	No. words per T-unit	
Reduced complexity of language	Reduced complexity of language	Not reported—assume it is reduced
% dependent clauses	% dependent clauses	
% nonfinite clauses	% nonfinite clauses	
No. clauses per T-unit		

Gleason et al. (1980) found similar results in their study using The Picture Story Test. Total output was reduced in Broca's but not in Wernicke's aphasic subjects. Complexity of language was reduced in both groups. Wernicke's aphasic subjects tended to concatenate sentences with "and" rather than to subordinate clauses with embedding.

Variables to control in discourse production are similar to those listed for conversation. Sufficient research is not available to list them hierarchically. Some examples of discourse are

> Narratives: Description of a place, person, event, experience
> Explanation of an event or proverb
> Story telling with or without a visual stimulus or auditory presentation
> Anecdotes

> Procedures: Telling how to do something,
> e.g., tie shoelaces, make a sandwich

> Expositions: Give a short speech about a particular subject
> Lecture on a particular topic

Description. These activities are designed to aid the aphasic patient's ability to retell or relate an experience or event. The patient is required to sequence logically a series of events or ideas and to express them orally. The sequence may vary in length and complexity of the topic being discussed.

Example. The aphasic patient relates a story that was heard on a news broadcast the previous evening, including three major ideas from the news report.

Chapter 9

Materials for Oral Expression

Area 1: Automatic Speech Series

Beginning Levels

Level 1

Stimuli. Items in series

Set A	Set B
1. counting	1. alphabet
2. days of week	2. months of year
3. greetings	3. poems

Procedure. The clinician orally provides the items in the series. A written form of the stimuli may also supplement the model. The patient is then required to produce the series in unison with the clinician.

Level 2

Stimuli. Items in series

Set A	Set B
1. counting	1. alphabet
2. days of week	2. months of year
3. greetings	3. poems

Procedure. The clinician orally produces the items in the series supplemented by a written form of the stimuli if facilitative. The first item in the series is then provided by the clinician and the patient is required to provide the remainder. The clinician supplies missing elements in the series as needed.

Level 3

Stimuli. Items in series

Set A	Set B
1. counting	1. alphabet
2. days of week	2. months of year
3. greetings	3. poems

Procedure. The clinician requests the patient to provide the elements in the series without an oral model or written stimuli.

Additional Levels

Additional levels may be developed by requiring the patient to use elements of automatic speech series in day-to-day conversation; for example, asking the patient what day it is or having the patient practice the use of greetings when entering the clinic.

Area 2: Phonological-Articulatory Production

Intermediate Levels

Level 1

Stimuli. Three syllable abstract words; grades 7 and 8 vocabulary

Set A	Set B
1. reluctant	1. persuasion
2. contradict	2. flattery
3. bravery	3. magnify
4. scarcity	4. tedious
5. radiance	5. dreadfully
6. magnitude	6. feverish
7. requisite	7. indignant
8. dividend	8. objective
9. modesty	9. repentance
10. disregard	10. exhaustion

Procedure. The clinician orally presents the stimuli, and the patient is required to produce each item correctly five times and use the word in a sentence.

Stimuli. Five to six syllable abstract words; grades 7 and 8 vocabulary

Set A	Set B
1. Presbyterian	1. authoritative
2. metropolitan	2. architectural
3. intolerable	3. unexpectedly
4. unreasonable	4. simultaneously
5. perpendicular	5. automatically
6. Christianity	6. indefinitely
7. administrative	7. denomination
8. realization	8. modification
9. insignificant	9. superiority
10. immortality	10. psychological

Procedure. The clinician orally presents the stimuli, and the patient is required to produce each item correctly five times.

Level 3

Stimuli. 8 to 10 syllable abstract word pairs; grades 7 and 8 vocabulary

Set A	Set B
1. beautifully intercepted	1. appalling realization
2. vigorously apprehended	2. sentimental adaptation
3. instinctively diplomatic	3. noticeable inconvenience
4. corresponding extravagance	4. negotiate indefinitely
5. overwhelming transformation	5. reluctantly apologize
6. enormously superstitious	6. monotonous deliberation
7. momentary interruption	7. administrative catastrophe
8. repeatedly humiliate	8. insignificant deficiency
9. automatically decompose	9. automatically apprehend
10. participate unexpectedly	10. experimental modification

Procedure. The clinician orally presents the stimuli, and the patient is required to produce each item correctly five times.

Additional Levels

Additional levels may be developed by increasing the length and grade level of the items and including them in more complicated contexts.

Area 3: Repetition

Intermediate-Advanced Levels

Level 1

Stimuli. 10 to 13 syllable sentences; grades 5 to 6 vocabulary

Set A

1. The pumpkins were advertised for Thanksgiving.
2. The bachelor is an extravagant escort.
3. Tablets were prescribed for his painful headache.
4. The hasty announcement was unexpected.
5. The chemist is an eminent scientist.
6. His popularity was shattered by the scandal.
7. We indulged ourselves with an incredible dessert.
8. The rumors provoked his resignation.
9. The substantial allowance was resented.
10. Let's congratulate her on her promotion.

Set B

1. The constable uncovered the conspiracy.
2. The manuscript is in the typewriter.
3. The baker modified the ingredients.
4. The surgeon was notified of the emergency.
5. The architect enlarged the nursery.
6. The publicity will prolong negotiations.
7. I promoted the ambitious undertaking.
8. She was embarrassed by his radical behavior.
9. Attendance at the celebration was dismal.
10. The aged preacher faltered during his sermon.

Procedure. The clinician auditorily presents a sentence, and the patient is required to imitate it.

Level 2

Stimuli. 10 to 13 syllable sentences; grades 9 to 12 vocabulary

Set A

1. The druggist's cologne is inexpensive.
2. The playwright was disheartened by the biography.
3. The arrogant celebrity was unpopular.
4. The administrator supervised the novice.
5. His disapproval affected the performer.

6. The animosity was misunderstood.
7. I abstained from the blueberries and champagne.
8. The streetcar narrowly eluded the collision.
9. There is an assortment of homemade doughnuts.
10. I agonized over your ruthless deception.

Set B

1. Oftentimes, we harmonize for relaxation.
2. The bootleggers will congregate in the barnyard.
3. A designer coordinated the salon.
4. Their reconciliation is miraculous.
5. The pedestrians are appalled by the peddlers.
6. Don't be disconcerted by all of the calories.
7. The dictator's memoirs were confiscated.
8. The landlady persevered with her housework.
9. Pneumonia is a pending complication.
10. The tornado devastated the courthouse.

Procedure. The clinician auditorily presents a sentence, and the patient is required to repeat it.

Level 3

Stimuli. 22 to 27 syllable sentences; grades 5 to 6 vocabulary

Set A

1. Her incredible determination effectively overwhelmed her shrewd competitors.
2. The preliminary recommendations of the superintendent were interpreted with caution.
3. The newcomers accumulated and cheerfully conversed in the picturesque surroundings.
4. His apprehension about the housekeeper was unfortunately interpreted as contempt.
5. The disagreeable producer fostered inevitable rebellion in the actress.
6. Unfortunately, there is significant controversy over the substantial inheritance.
7. Her apprehension about his conservative leadership dominated the proceedings.
8. The exquisite dancers were congratulated on their ambitious undertaking.
9. I invariably commend her on her popularity as a fantastic hostess.
10. Subsequently, the concerned landlord cooperated with the efficient inspector.

Set B

1. The millionaire's formidable housekeeper angrily rebuked the offensive butler.
2. Ordinarily, the grocer successfully promoted the poultry, bacon, and sausages.
3. The affectionate inscription on the bracelet reassured her about their relationship.
4. The musician was congratulated on his accomplishments with an enthusiastic demonstration.
5. The proprietor intervened in the unnecessary disturbance related to alcohol.
6. Because of her unpleasant temperament, the volunteer was excluded from the banquet.
7. The millionaire circulated at the fashionable reception.
8. Unfortunately, there was outstanding speculation over the signature on the document.
9. The shoemaker exaggerated to the barber about his misfortune after the explosion.
10. The controversy over the publication was anticipated by the clergyman.

Procedure. The clinician auditorily presents a sentence, and the patient is required to repeat it.

Additional Levels

Additional levels may be developed by manipulating variables such as immediacy of the response.

Area 4: Oral Reading

The following material was designed for patients demonstrating deep dyslexia. Other parameters would need to be altered for those with pure alexia, surface dyslexia, or phonological dyslexia.

Intermediate Levels

Level 1

Stimuli. Content words; high imageability; grades 5 to 8 vocabulary

Set A	Set B
1. partridge	1. balloon
2. terrace	2. abdomen

‌‍‌‌‍‌

3.	bologna	3.	gardener
4.	scissors	4.	revolver
5.	camera	5.	appliance
6.	upstairs	6.	pedestal
7.	freckle	7.	trumpet
8.	nursery	8.	shingle
9.	mosquito	9.	mushroom
10.	rainbow	10.	donkey

Procedure. A printed word is presented to the patient, who is required to read it aloud.

Level 2

Stimuli. Content words; high imageability; grades 9 to 12 vocabulary

Set A   **Set B**

1.	postman	1.	bedside
2.	tablecloth	2.	custard
3.	garbage	3.	vulture
4.	vacuum	4.	scallop
5.	diploma	5.	thimble
6.	moccasin	6.	chateau
7.	cartoon	7.	emblem
8.	lipstick	8.	organist
9.	funnel	9.	knuckle
10.	streamer	10.	diploma

Procedure. A printed word is presented to the patient, who is required to read it aloud.

Level 3

Stimuli. Content words; low imageability; grades 5 to 8 vocabulary

Set A   **Set B**

1.	secrecy	1.	grammar
2.	manhood	2.	maturity
3.	fiction	3.	regime
4.	episode	4.	duration
5.	integrity	5.	treason
6.	premise	6.	courtesy
7.	nonsense	7.	proverb
8.	downfall	8.	foresight

9. chivalry	9. symptom
10. trustee	10. omission

Procedure. A printed word is presented to the patient, who is required to read it aloud.

Additional Levels

Additional levels may be developing by including adjectives, verbs, function words, and nonwords. The length of the stimuli could be increased by using the words in phrases and sentences.

Area 5: Oral Spelling

The following material was designed for patients demonstrating surface dyslexia. Other parameters would need to be altered for those with deep dyslexia.

Intermediate to Advanced Levels

Level 1

Stimuli. 4 to 6 letter words; grades 9 to 12 vocabulary; regular spelling

Set A	Set B
1. pact	1. probe
2. fang	2. haze
3. munch	3. dike
4. stove	4. sheaf
5. needy	5. thinly
6. verb	6. zest
7. shrank	7. slat
8. gill	8. caste
9. clod	9. vista
10. wick	10. mink

Procedure. The clinician auditorily presents a word, and the patient is required to spell it orally.

Level 2

Stimuli. 4 to 6 letter words; grades 9 to 12 vocabulary; irregular spelling

Set A	Set B
1. gnat	1. eunuch
2. balk	2. beau
3. knack	3. gauge
4. chintz	4. czar
5. abyss	5. ensign
6. lynch	6. prism
7. satyr	7. watt
8. · scythe	8. seethe
9. niche·	9. balmy
10. deign	10. numb

Procedure. The clinician auditorily presents a word, and the patient is required to spell it orally. Words with dual spellings may be provided in the context of a sentence.

Level 3

Stimuli. 9 to 10 letter words; grades 9 to 12 vocabulary; regular spelling

Set A	Set B
1. prevailing	1. paramount
2. roundabout	2. blameless
3. inability	3. transcript
4. waistcoat	4. cultivated
5. impediment	5. dormitory
6. frankness	6. servitude
7. suffocate	7. benevolent
8. threescore	8. hundredth
9. attainment	9. millstone
10. preaching	10. impending

Procedure. The clinician auditorily presents a word and the patient is required to spell it orally.

Additional Levels

Additional levels may be developed by increasing the word length. By altering word type, for example, concrete-abstract, content-functor, along with incorporating irregularly spelled words, difficulty level may be increased.

Area 6: Word Retrieval or Anomia

Advanced Levels

Level 1

Stimuli. Sentences to elicit; nouns; grades 9 to 12 vocabulary

Set A

1. The artist put several colors on his _____ . (palette)
2. People on diets have to count their _____ . (calories)
3. The Indians used to wear _____ on their feet. (moccasins)
4. When the baby smiled, two tiny _____ appeared on her cheeks. (dimples)
5. The race in which runners pass batons to each other is called a _____ . (relay)
6. The country situated near Australia is _____ . (New Zealand)
7. The string instrument that is slightly larger than a violin is a _____ . (viola)
8. Because the road was under construction, we had to take a _____ . (detour)
9. The woman covered the table with a pretty _____ . (tablecloth)
10. Most of the players are over six feet tall in the game of _____ . (basketball)

Set B

1. Their portrait was taken by a professional _____ . (photographer)
2. For protection, the prime minister was surrounded by his _____ . (bodyguards)
3. He made a generous _____ to his favorite charity. (donation)
4. They raked up the leaves and burned them in a _____ . (bonfire)
5. After the defense questioned him, the man was questioned by the _____ . (prosecution)
6. After receiving a standing ovation, the musician gave an _____. (encore)
7. In the winter, trappers wear _____ to walk in the bush. (snowshoes)
8. A snakelike creature that lives in the water is the _____ . (eel)
9. He received a second _____ that his books were overdue. (reminder)
10. The faulty wiring was repaired by the _____ . (electrician)

Procedure. The names of three types of cues that have been determined effective for the patient are placed on written cards. The patient, when unable to complete the sentence, is required to ask the clinician for a given type of cue. The sentence may be presented either auditorily or visually for completion. If the patient provides an appropriate word of a lower vocabulary level, she or he is encouraged to think of a synonym. However, the response would be considered correct.

Level 2

Stimuli. Sentences to elicit; nouns; grades 9 to 12 vocabulary

Set A

1. A true _____ is interested in how he plays, not if he wins. (sportsman)
2. A person who hoards all of his money is called a _____ . (miser)
3. If you collect antiques, a good place to look is a country _____ . (auction)
4. The hunters set out their duck _____ . (decoys)
5. Who won the race between the _____ and the hare? (tortoise)
6. When you have surgery, you are usually given a general _____ . (anaesthetic)
7. The animal with a ringed tail and masked face is the _____ . (raccoon)
8. The reproduction was so good, even the experts couldn't tell that it was a _____ . (fake)
9. The offices were cleaned by the night _____ . (janitor)
10. The employee cashed his _____ at the bank. (check)

Set B

1. He felt that his constant fatigue was not due to sickness but rather to _____ . (boredom)
2. Some politicians are more interested in power and _____ than in their constituents. (prestige)
3. He watched the birds with a pair of _____ . (binoculars)
4. On a scale of one to ten, the flowers were given a _____ of seven. (rating)
5. Three policemen received awards for their acts of _____ . (bravery)
6. He ate the apple right down to the _____ . (core)
7. At Christmas, couples kiss under the _____ . (mistletoe)

8. Soon after the man jumped out of the plane, his _____ opened. (parachute)
9. The car could not drive up the icy hill because it didn't have enough _____ . (traction)
10. In medieval times, the king was entertained by the court _____ . (jester)

Procedure. The names of three types of cues that have been determined effective for the patient are placed on written cards. When the patient is unable to complete the sentence, the clinician points to one of the cards and requests that the patient orally produce the cue. The remaining cues are attempted if success is not achieved on the first trial.

Level 3

Stimuli. Sentences to elicit; nouns; grades 9 to 12 vocabulary

Set A

1. Next month, I will be attending my brother's _____ from the university. (graduation)
2. On Remembrance Day, we wear a _____ on our lapel. (poppy)
3. In September, I enjoy watching _____ for the new television season. (previews)
4. The judge walked back to his chambers in the _____ . (courthouse)
5. After a storm on the ocean, a lot of _____ washes up on the beach. (driftwood)
6. At the end of the prayer, the congregation all said _____ . (amen)
7. He owns his own business, although it is part of a chain, because he has purchased the _____ . (franchise)
8. He hurried home to see the final _____ of the program for the season. (episode)
9. After the plane crash, they found only one _____ . (survivor)
10. The letters *RR* are an _____ for rural route. (abbreviation)

Set B

1. In the comic strips, "Snoopy" is the name of a _____ dog. (beagle)
2. Red Skelton is the name of a famous _____ . (comedian)
3. The pupil removed the pencil marks from his sheet with an _____ . (eraser)
4. I took my watch to the _____ for repair. (jeweler)
5. Every Tuesday morning our _____ is collected. (garbage)

6. The employer interviewed several _____ for the position. (applicants)
7. The explosion was believed to be caused by _____ . (dynamite)
8. A tall building is called a _____ . (skyscraper)
9. The bride and groom were toasted with _____ . (champagne)
10. There has been a long-standing _____ between the competitors. (rivalry)

Procedure. The names of three types of cues that have been determined effective for the patient are placed on written cards. The patient is required to use the cues without prompting when she or he fails to spontaneously complete a sentence.

Additional Levels

Additional levels may be developed by including stimuli from other word classes. The activity level may also be made more difficult by incorporating the use of cueing in conversational speech.

Area 7: Oral Formulation

Intermediate-Advanced Levels

Stimuli. Sentences to elicit; formulation of the passive transformation

Set A

1. The woman is making the bed.
    What is happening to the bed? Tell me about the bed.
    Response: The bed is being made by the woman.
2. The man is painting the window.
    What is happening to the window? Tell me about the window.
    Response: The window is being painted by the man.
3. My son is driving the truck.
    What is happening to the truck? Tell me about the truck.
    Response: The truck is being driven by my son.
4. The girl is sweeping the floor.
    What is happening to the floor? Tell me about the floor.
    Response: The floor is being swept by the girl.
5. The boxer is hitting the bag.
    What is happening to the bag? Tell me about the bag.
    Response: The bag is being hit by the boxer.
6. My neighbor is raking leaves.
    What is happening to the leaves? Tell me about the leaves.
    Response: The leaves are being raked by my neighbor.

7. The baker is making a cake.
    What is happening to the cake? Tell me about the cake.
    Response: The cake is being made by the baker.
8. Father is drinking water.
    What is happening to the water? Tell me about the water.
    Response: The water is being drunk by father.
9. The gardener is cutting the grass.
    What is happening to the grass? Tell me about the grass.
    Response: The grass is being cut by the gardener.
10. The children are watching television.
    What is happening to the television? Tell me about the television.
    Response: The television is being watched by the children.

Set B

1. The dog is chewing his bone.
    What is happening to the bone? Tell me about the bone.
    Response: The bone is being chewed by the dog.
2. The mechanic is fixing the car.
    What is happening to the car? Tell me about the car.
    Response: The car is being fixed by the mechanic.
3. My aunt is knitting a sweater.
    What is happening to the sweater? Tell me about the sweater.·
    Response: The sweater is being knit by my aunt.
4. The teacher is marking papers.
    What is happening to the papers? Tell me about the papers.
    Response: The papers are being marked by the teacher.
5. The secretary is typing a letter.
    What is happening to the letter? Tell me about the letter.
    Response: The letter is being typed by the secretary.
6. The nurse is giving pills.
    What is happening to the pills? Tell me about the pills.
    Response: The pills are being given by the nurse.
7. The mailman is delivering mail.
    What is happening to the mail? Tell me about the mail.
    Response: The mail is being delivered by the mailman.
8. The waiter is pouring the wine.
    What is happening to the wine? Tell me about the wine.
    Response: The wine is being poured by the waiter.
9. The guest is washing dishes.
    What is happening to the dishes? Tell me about the dishes.
    Response: The dishes are being washed by the guest.

10. The carpenter is cutting the wood.
     What is happening to the wood? Tell me about the wood.
     Response: The wood is being cut by the carpenter.

Procedure. The clinician auditorily presents a statement followed by a question, a statement, or both to elicit formulation of a passive transformation. The stimuli may be supplemented by pictures.

Level 2

Stimuli. Sentences to elicit formulation of relative clauses that modify nouns used as objects of verbs or prepositions.

Set A

1. a. The man stood beside the train.
    b. The train was leaving.
    Response: The man stood beside the train that was leaving.
2. a. The child knocked down the blind.
    b. The blind was broken.
    Response: The child knocked down the blind, which was broken.
3. a. The woman went to the doctor.
    b. The doctor was a friend.
    Response: The woman went to the doctor who was a friend.
4. a. I talked to the girl.
    b. The girl returned from Mexico.
    Response: I talked to the girl who returned from Mexico.
5. a. His cousin went to the baseball game.
    b. The game was rained out.
    Response: His cousin went to the baseball game that was rained out.
6. a. His friends are in the library.
    b. The library is closing.
    Response: His friends are in the library, which is closing.
7. a. The students were upset about the exam.
    b. The exam was long.
    Response: The students were upset about the exam, which was long.
8. a. Mother is calling the plumber.
    b. The plumber is late.
    Response: Mother is calling the plumber, who is late.
9. a. The hitchhiker was near the city.
    b. The city was a mile away.
    Response: The hitchhiker was near the city, which was a mile away.

10. a. The cat is sitting on the table.
     b. The table is an antique.
     Response: The cat is sitting on the table that is an antique.

Set B

1. a. The car was stalled on the road.
    b. The road was very busy.
    Response: The car was stalled on the road that was very busy.
2. a. We invited our co-workers.
    b. Our co-workers are all women.
    Response: We invited our co-workers, who are all women.
3. a. The team defeated the champions.
    b. The champions were poor losers.
    Response: The team defeated the champions, who were poor losers.
4. a. The newsboy delivered the paper.
    b. The paper is on the porch.
    Response: The newsboy delivered the paper, which is on the porch.
5. a. The bus hit the pedestrian.
    b. The pedestrian was crossing the street.
    Response: The bus hit the pedestrian who was crossing the street.
6. a. The men ate dinner at a restaurant.
    b. The restaurant was downtown.
    Response: The men ate dinner at a restaurant that was downtown.
7. a. The light is on in the attic.
    b. The attic is usually dark.
    Response: The light is on in the attic, which is usually dark.
8. a. The housekeeper prepares dinner.
    b. Dinner is never late.
    Response: The housekeeper prepares dinner, which is never late.
9. a. She is waiting with her escort.
    b. Her escort is a good dancer.
    Response: She is waiting with her escort, who is a good dancer.
10. a. The druggist sells magazines.
     b. The magazines are in the third aisle.
     Response: The druggist sells magazines, which are in the third
              aisle.

Procedure. The clinician auditorily presents two sentences for the patient to combine and orally produce. A visual presentation method is also possible.

Level 3

Stimuli. Sentences to elicit formulation of relative clauses used as adverbials.

Set A

1. a. Yesterday was the day.
    b. He accepted the position.
    When did he accept the position?
    Response: Yesterday was the day when he accepted the position.
2. a. Mr. Jones was upset.
    b. He heard about the news.
    When was Mr. Jones upset?
    Response: Mr. Jones was upset when he heard about the news.
3. a. New York is a city.
    b. You can find excitement there.
    What kind of a city is New York?
    Response: New York is a city where you can find excitement.
4. a. The plant grows well in the window.
    b. The sun shines there.
    Where does the plant grow well?
    Response: The plant grows well in the window where the sun shines.
5. a. It was very late.
    b. I finally got to sleep.
    When did I get to sleep?
    Response: It was very late when I finally got to sleep.
6. a. They took the lock off the door.
    b. It didn't work.
    When did they take the lock off the door?
    Response: They took the lock off the door when it didn't work.
7. a. The woman on the bus was hurt.
    b. The bus stopped suddenly.
    When was the woman on the bus hurt?
    Response: The woman on the bus was hurt when it stopped suddenly.
8. a. Tomorrow we will go to the lake.
    b. The swimming is good at the lake.
    Where will we go tomorrow?
    Response: Tomorrow we will go to the lake, where the swimming is good.

9. a. John is in the waiting room.
    b. The magazines are kept in the waiting room.
    Where is John?
    Response: John is in the waiting room, where the magazines are
        kept.
10. a. He cleaned the carpet.
    b. The carpet was dirty.
    When did he clean the carpet?
    Response: He cleaned the carpet when it was dirty.

Set B

1. a. His wife came to the hospital.
    b. She heard of the accident.
    When did his wife come to the hospital?
    Response: His wife came to the hospital when she heard of the
        accident.
2. a. The worker went to the unemployment office.
    b. He was looking for a job.
    When did the worker go to the unemployment office?
    Response: The worker went to the unemployment office when he was
        looking for a job.
3. a. The children played in the backyard.
    b. There was more room in the backyard.
    Where did the children play?
    Response: The children played in the backyard where there was
        more room.
4. a. The artist is painting in his studio.
    b. He has privacy in his studio.
    Where does the artist paint?
    Response: The artist paints in his studio, where he has privacy.
5. a. The lawyer called the judge.
    b. The judge was sympathetic.
    Who did the lawyer call?
    Response: The lawyer called the judge, who was sympathetic.
6. a. The investigator solved the case.
    b. The case was five years old.
    When did the investigator solve the case?
    Response: The investigator solved the case when it was five
        years old.
7. a. The tourist left her camera on the beach.
    b. There were many people on the beach.
    Where did the tourist leave her camera?
    Response: The tourist left her camera on the beach where there were
        many people.

8. a. The trucker stopped at the roadside.
   b. He saw an accident.
   When did the trucker stop at the roadside?
   Response: The trucker stopped at the roadside when he saw an
   accident.
9. a. The couple attended the theater.
   b. The theater was renovated.
   When did the couple attend the theater?
   Response: The couple attended the theater when it was renovated.
10. a. The policeman rushed to the hotel.
    b. There was a brawl at the hotel.
    Where did the policeman rush?
    Response: The policeman rushed to the hotel where there was a
    brawl.

Procedure. The clinician auditorily presents two sentences for the
patient to combine and orally produce. A visual presentation method is
also possible.

Additional Levels

Additional levels may be developed by introducing more difficult sentence
structures, such as yes-no questions.

Area 8: Conversation

Beginning Levels

Level 1

Stimuli. Familiar topics with a familiar person in a familiar setting

Set A	**Set B**
Activities of the patient's family members	A trip that the patient has taken

Procedure. The clinician engages the patient in conversation about a
familiar topic for 5 minutes, in the clinic.

Level 2

Stimuli. Less familiar topics with a familiar person in a familiar setting

Set A	**Set B**
A current event with which the patient is only partially familiar	A recreational activity in which the patient has never engaged

Procedure. The clinician engages the patient in conversation about a less familiar topic for 5 minutes, in the clinic.

Level 3

Stimuli. Familiar topics with an unfamiliar speaker in a familiar setting

Set A	Set B
Hobby or recreational activity of the patient	The patient's work

Procedure. An unfamiliar person engages the patient in a conversation about a familiar topic for 5 minutes, in the clinic.

Additional Levels

Additional levels may be developed by changing the setting to a less familiar one and increasing the number of participants in the conversation.

Area 9: Discourse

Beginning Levels

Level 1

Stimuli. Narratives

Set A	Set B
Retelling of a newspaper article	Retelling of a television program

Procedure. The patient is required to orally provide a narrative about material read, heard, or viewed.

Level 2

Stimuli. Procedures

Set A	Set B
Steps involved in planning a dinner party	Steps involved in organizing a garage sale

Procedure. The patient is required to orally outline steps involved in certain activities.

Level 3

Stimuli. Expository

Set A

Views on gun control

Set B

Views on the relationship
between religion and politics

Procedure. The patient is required to orally provide a short speech about a particular subject matter.

Additional Levels

Additional levels may be developed by increasing the amount of detail required in the patient's discourse activities.

Chapter 10

Treatment for Graphic Expression

Graphic expression refers to the expression of messages utilizing a written form of output, usually graphemes (letters), although drawings or typing movements could also be used. As such, writing involves the complex interaction among several systems—the limb motor system, the linguistic system, and feedback from sensory systems, such as the visual and kinesthetic.

Writing disorders, often referred to by the terms agraphia or dysgraphia, form part of the symptom complex of aphasia. Although they may differ in type and severity for patients, writing is generally the most severely impaired of the language modalities (Henri, 1973; Schuell et al., 1964; among others), but there are exceptions to this reported in the literature (Basso, Taborelli, and Vignolo, 1978; Bub and Kertesz, 1982b; Hier and Mohr, 1977). Agraphia, on the other hand, as a general term that refers to impaired writing due to acquired brain damage, describes writing disorders consisting of clinically different behaviors. Not all agraphias are alike, and it is important to describe their differences and similarities to assist the clinician in providing appropriate treatment.

As is the case for reading, not all aphasic patients will utilize writing abilities extensively, a situation that also applies to normal individuals (Chédru and Geschwind, 1972). The amount and nature of treatment work for this modality, therefore, will be influenced by the patient's needs and interests as well as education level and premorbid proficiency. It is important to differentiate errors characteristic of aphasia from those associated with a low educational level (Keenan and Brassell, 1972). Our previous comments (Chapter 4) on literacy and the appropriateness of treatment are also relevant here.

It has often been written that aphasic patients write as they speak. There is certainly some clinical validity to this statement. Speech-language pathologists have all seen the parallels between the agrammatic speech and writing of some Broca's aphasic patients and the copious jargon speech and writing of some Wernicke's individuals. However, since there are differences in the spoken and written language of normal adults, at least in college students, it is well to remember that these may also emerge in the aphasic patient (Gibson, Gruner, Kibler, and Kelly, 1966).

Since disorders in graphic expression have been studied extensively only within recent years, researchers have just started to delineate various subtypes. Although more is being learned about agraphia and its association with aphasia and other neurological impairments, this has precipitated numerous ways of classifying agraphia, a situation that can be confusing to readers (see Fig. 1–10). One classification system has made the distinction between agraphia occurring alone (pure agraphia) or in concert with other symptoms, leading to terms such as alexia with agraphia, aphasic agraphia, and apractic agraphia. Another classification dichotomized agraphia into motor and linguistic types (affecting spelling and meaning). A third differentiation was made according to the neuroanatomical correlates of the writing disturbance, producing dominant frontal (anterior) agraphia, dominant parietal-temporal (posterior) agraphia, and nondominant agraphia (Benson, 1979a). More recently

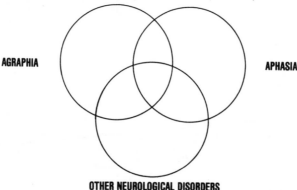

Figure 10–1. This figure indicates the overlapping nature of aphasic written language disorders, agraphic disorders, and written language problems of other neurologically based disorders.

researchers have divided the agraphias according to their neuro-psychological correlates, producing terms such as phonological agraphia, lexical agraphia, and semantic agraphia. (For a more complete review of neuropsychological descriptions of writing, the reader is referred to Ellis, 1982, and Margolin, 1984.)

The relationship between aphasia and agraphia parallels that between aphasia and alexia. Writing disturbances are part and parcel of aphasia, and therefore all aphasic individuals could be termed agraphic. However, in the context of aphasia, the term usually emphasizes a particular type of writing disturbance, such as phonological agraphia, rather than the presence of a disturbance. Agraphias can occur in the absence of aphasia, such as in acute confusional states (Chédru and Geschwind, 1972), or in isolation (e.g., pure agraphia). Agraphias can also be present in aphasic patients although not part of the aphasia per se (e.g., apractic agraphia).

TYPES OF GRAPHIC EXPRESSION DEFICITS

Motor Production and Motor Planning Deficits

Some aphasic patients will have difficulty writing because of motor problems. These can arise in the execution stage of graphic or graphemic production due to paresis of the writing hand. The consequence of this impairment is the distorted production of graphemes, which may make the writing difficult to read.

A common occurrence is aphasia is the presence of right-sided hemiplegia. Since the hand movements necessary to produce handwriting are absent, writing is usually tested in the nondominant hand. Writing with this hand has reportedly been impaired, particularly in Broca's aphasic patients, beyond the level expected for the use of the nonpreferred hand (Benson, 1979a). The handwriting is often poor mechanically, with large, poorly formed letters even in copying. Researchers have explained this disturbance on the basis of a sympathetic dyspraxia. The mechanical difficulties are frequently associated with linguistic errors in writing, such as spelling errors and agrammatic output. Some refer to this constellation of symptoms as callosal dysgraphia although it is not clear whether the dysgraphia results from apraxia or whether it arises from a disconnection of the left hand from the language area (Albert, Goodglass, Helm, Rubens, and Alexander, 1981).

Using a prosthetic device that would allow the hemiplegic hand to write has revealed that at least some aphasic patients have superior writing with this hand than with the nonhemiplegic left hand (Brown, Leader, and Blum, 1983; Leischner, 1983). These patients wrote better to dictation and copied better on their hemiplegic side. Since Brown and co-workers' three patients were able to perform cross-modal transfer tasks, such as writing the name of an object with the right hand that had been palpated with the left hand, they discounted the disconnection syndrome explanation for the poor performance of the left hand. Brown and colleagues (1983) postulated that the hemiplegic writing used a different muscle system, one subserving axial and proximal movement, which had access to "submerged levels in language in the damaged (or intact?) hemsphere" (p. 213).

Although impaired motor production is usually the effect of noncortical lesions, syntactic writing problems were reported by Ferguson and Boller (1977) in three patients with motor speech disorders. Since the motor functioning of the limbs was also involved, problems with the mechanics of writing might be expected. However, the two ALS patients and the palilalic patient demonstrated spelling, syntactic, and perseverative errors. The authors postulated an "efferent motor agraphia," with the syntactic problems resulting from disturbed feedback from both the speech and hand movement systems.

In order to produce accurate handwriting, a person must select the appropriate graphemic motor patterns that correspond to the letters composing a word. If these motor patterns are damaged or are inaccessible, the aphasic patient will not produce the correct graphemes. Apractic agraphia, sometimes referred to as parietal agraphia, has frequently been found associated with parietal lobe lesions (Albert et al., 1981; Marcie and Hécaen, 1979). The apractic agraphic patient produces a meaningless scrawl because he or she cannot form the correct graphemes (Geschwind and Kaplan, 1962; Margolin and Binder, 1984; Marcie and Hécaen, 1979; Roeltgen and Heilman, 1983). Most patients copy much better than they write to dictation. Using Ellis's (1982) model of writing, these patients have their major deficit at the graphic motor pattern component. It is at this stage that the subject must use the long-term memory store of graphemic motor patterns, which specify the relative size and sequence of letter strokes. By using the copying behavior of a patient with apractic agraphia, Margolin and Binder (1984) were able to analyze at least some of the problems leading to his illegible handwriting. This patient selected the wrong letter element (e.g., a loop rather than a horizontal line in ε versus G), put an element in the wrong spatial position (e.g., horizontal bar is incorrectly placed in ε versus G), showed incorrect rotation (e.g., ς versus S), repeated appropriate strokes (e.g., m versus m), and demonstrated inappropriate orientation (e.g., Γ versus M). Of course, in spontaneous writing when the target is not known, such an analysis may not be possible.

Problems with the Physical Letter Code

In some patients spelling is better in one output modality than another. For example, Kinsbourne and Rosenfeld (1974) and Rothi and Heilman (1981) reported cases of alexia with agraphia in which oral spelling was spared relative to written spelling. Rothi and Heilman's patient's auditory comprehension and repetition were excellent, fluency was normal with only slightly reduced spontaneous speech, and a mild anomia was present. He was able to read simple words but not sentences. He made errors in writing words spontaneously and to dictation, producing well-formed but incorrect graphemes. His performance on anagrams (81 percent) was almost twice that for written spelling (41 percent). He was also able to name words spelled orally to him. This pattern of performance suggested that the patient could recognize and produce letter names and could recognize but not construct the corresponding graphemes. Rothi and Heilman (1981) hypothesized that the graphemic area, which is responsible for distinguishing the features of graphemes and for guiding motor programming of grapheme production, was destroyed or disconnected from the area of visual word images, that is, the orthographic code. Margolin (1984) had a similar explanation of a disconnection between the physical letter code and the graphic motor patterns or a problem with the motor patterns themselves. This constituted what they termed a transitional agraphia.

Phonemic-Graphemic Conversion and Lexical Processing Deficits

Through studying the reading process and through the observation that the writing disturbances of aphasic individuals were not always similar, detailed investigations of agraphia revealed at least two disturbances in the writing process that affected spelling. Other writing deficits might also be present but the focus was on single-word spelling and the error types observed.

For patients who could write to dictation regular and irregularly spelled words but not nonwords (e.g., gintch), researchers concluded that the primary deficit lay in difficulties with phonemic-graphemic conversion. The patients could hear the word and repeat it accurately but could not write the word. This type of agraphia has most commonly been referred to as phonological agraphia or nonlexical agraphia (Margolin, 1984; Shallice, 1981). Familiar words, whether spelled regularly (phonetically, e.g., hat) or irregularly (nonphonetically, e.g., cough), may be accessed from the semantic system and directly transcoded into graphemic form. The phonemic-graphemic route is not involved. However, this semantic route does not apply to nonwords, as the only way they can be spelled is via phonemic-graphemic conversion. In spelling, these patients make several types of errors: derivational errors in which the written word is a derivation of the target (e.g., magical/magician), structural errors in which the patient's response is structurally similar to the target (e.g., sanity/sanitation) and incorrect spelling (e.g., folow/follow) (Bub and Kertesz, 1982b).

Type of aphasia present in the reported cases has varied. Both cases reported by Bub and Kertesz (1982a, 1982b) and two in the Roeltgen, Sevush, and Heilman series (1983) demonstrated Broca's aphasia. Three Wernicke's patients (Hier and Mohr, 1977; Roeltgen et al., 1983) as well as one almost completely resolved conduction aphasic patient (Shallice, 1981) have also presented with this spelling difficulty. As might be expected, their spoken language and other features of the aphasia were dissimilar and consistent with their type classification and locus of lesion. Roeltgen and colleagues (1983) have postulated that the lesion responsible for phonological agraphia lies in the supramarginal gyrus.

When symptoms of phonological agraphia occur in association with poorer spelling of abstract than concrete words, poorer spelling of functor versus content words, and poorer spelling of verbs than nouns, this has been referred to as deep agraphia (Bub and Kertesz, 1982a). This term was coined because of the similarities between the writing disturbance and reading problems (deep dyslexia).

When the semantic route to spelling words is impaired and the patient tries to spell words phonetically, the term lexical or semantic agraphia has been applied. These aphasic patients show a discrepancy in their spelling of regular (phonetic) and irregular (nonphonetic) words. They can spell nonwords because they have retained their ability to convert phonemes to graphemes and use precisely this approach to spelling. These patients copy well because their spelling errors are phonologically based, that is, they tend to spell the word as it sounds (e.g., fone/phone; mischef/mischief) (Beauvois and Dérouesné, 1981; Roeltgen and Heilman, 1984; Roeltgen, Rothi, and Heilman, 1982).

Patients with lexical agraphia generally demonstrate mild anomic or Wernicke's aphasia (Roeltgen and Heilman, 1984) although Beauvois and Dérouesné (1981) reported their patient revealed only phonological alexia without impairment of auditory comprehension and oral expression. The lesion thought to be responsible for lexical agraphia is in the angular gyrus (Roeltgen and Heilman, 1984).

Group design studies investigating spelling may have shown different results because of the heterogeneity of the dysgraphic problems seen in the patients (Friederici, Schoenle, and Goodglass, 1981; Langmore and Canter, 1983; Wapner and Gardner, 1979). These patients were grouped according to site of lesion (Wapner and Gardner, 1979) or to type of aphasia

(Friederici et al., 1981; Langmore and Canter, 1983). For example, Frie-derici and associates (1981) found two patterns among their Broca's patients, whereas Langmore and Canter (1983) found homogeneity. All their Broca's aphasic patients made many visually based errors and few phonically based ones. Wapner and Gardner's (1979) finding that anterior lesion patients used a strategy of "spell it as it looks" (phonological agra-phia) and posterior lesion patients used "spell it as it sounds" (lexical agraphia) appears to oversimplify the issue, given the recent material that associates both phonological and lexical agraphia with posterior lesions, supramarginal gyrus in the first case and angular gyrus in the second (Roeltgen and Heilman, 1984). The treatment guidelines outlined in this chapter take advantage of the new research on writing deficits to assist the clinician to design treatment specific to the deficits determined during assessment procedures.

Semantic-Syntactic Linguistic Processing Deficits

Writing, of course, is not restricted to copying and spelling single words. As with oral expression, words must be retrieved from long-term memory and arranged in sequence to produce meaningful written grammatical struc-tures, phrases, or sentences. Sentences are also arranged in larger units to produce discourse, such as narrative and procedural discourse.

Because the semantic-syntactic processing problems differ across types of aphasia these differences are reflected in the graphic expression modality as they were in the oral expression modality. The Broca's aphasic group shows limited written output characterized by agrammatism. There is a predominance of substantive words and the number of words in each run is small. Usually writing is more impaired than speaking and often more resistant to recovery (Benson, 1979a; Kaplan and Goodglass, 1981; Ulatowska, Baker, and Freedman-Stern, 1979). The written output of the transcortical motor aphasic group is limited. The patient may be able to manage short responsive writing, although longer material and narratives are impossible. When able to produce runs of words, they are agrammatic (Benson, 1979a). In global aphasia, writing is severely disturbed and fre-quently patients write nothing or may attempt only their name.

The writing of Wernicke's aphasic patients is often described as fluent and paragraphic (contains paraphasias). Although these patients write slowly and are reduced in output by comparison to their normal counter-parts (Freedman-Stern, Ulatowska, Baker, and Delacoste, 1984) they do not stuggle to form graphemes. Their runs of words are shorter than in speech and contain paraphasic substitutions and perhaps neologisms (Benson, 1979a). They tend to use vague referents, giving their writing an empty quality (Ulatowska et al., 1979). They frequently combine words in paragrammatic sentence forms, although their shorter runs tend to be more coherent (Goodglass and Hunter, 1970; Kaplan and Goodglass, 1981). Conduction aphasic patients also demonstrate impaired writing, with the degree of impairment seemingly dependent on the location and size of the lesion. Their writing is easily produced (fluent) and the graphemes are well formed. In grammatical structures, they may interchange, misplace, or omit words (Benson, 1979a). Their writing problems increase as the units progress in complexity. Writing may or may not be disturbed in anomic aphasia. The spelling deficits often associated with this type of aphasia (lexical agraphia) have been described, and Benson (1979a) reports that anomic aphasia may be associated with the syndrome of alexia with agraphia. Both are generally associated with lesions in the angular gyrus. Writing is defective in transcortical sensory aphasia, being characterized by paraphasias and fluent form. It is similar to the written output of the Wernicke's aphasic group (Benson, 1979a).

Nonaphasic Agraphias

It is neither the intention of nor is it within the scope of this chapter to review all the agraphias. However, familiarity with two additional types is important for the clinician.

Pure Agraphia

This refers to an isolated writing disturbance, one that occurs without other language impairments. It is a rare syndrome and researchers have not reached consensus about it. Chédru and Geschwind (1972) elaborated on the shortcomings of the reports of pure agraphia with focal lesions and contended that the same symptoms can be produced by diffuse brain dysfunction, as in acute confusional states. Some researchers associate pure agraphia with a frontal lesion at the foot of the second frontal convolution (Exner's area). However, others have described pure agraphia associated with parietal lesions (Albert et al., 1981; Hécaen and Albert, 1978; Kaplan and Goodglass, 1981; Marcie and Hécaen, 1979).

Spatial Agraphia

With nondominant lesions, usually right-hemisphere lesions, patients show disturbed spatial organization of their writing (Albert et al., 1981; Benson, 1979a; Hécaen and Albert, 1978; Marcie and Hécaen, 1979). Characteristics include a wide left margin on the page, reiteration of components of letters or complete letters themselves, and written lines deviating upward from the horizontal plane. Benson (1979) also noted an increase in the size of the writing with subsequent lines. This type of agraphia is mechanical in nature, with the semantic, syntactic, and word selection linguistic elements preserved. Spatial agraphia has been associated with right parietotempero-occipital lesions that result in a visuospatial impairment.

GUIDELINES FOR GRAPHIC EXPRESSION TREATMENT

The LOT treatment guidelines for graphic expression have been divided into three major categories: (1) those focusing on the recall, motor production, or both of graphic or graphemic patterns, (2) those emphasizing the spelling of single words, and (3) those requiring semantic-syntactic linguistic processing. Because any given aphasic patient may exhibit problems in more than one of these categories, treatment may occur concurrently in them. The areas within each category, however, are arranged according to increasing difficulty.

The activities in Areas 1 and 2 (see Chapter 1) focus on establishing or reactivating motor engrams or patterns for production. Area 1 utilizes graphic motor patterns, whereas Area 2 focuses on graphemic motor patterns. Some patients who do not demonstrate a constructional apraxia (drawing apraxia) may bypass Area 1. Others may benefit from treatment here, as witnessed by the success of some global aphasic patients with Visual Action Therapy (Helm and Benson, 1978; Helm-Estabrooks et al., 1982).

Area 3 requires the recall of graphemic motor patterns although in highly overlearned contexts, such as the patient's name, address, the alphabet, and elementary number series. The highly overlearned aspect of these may override the requirement of the recall of graphemic motor patterns and make this area no more difficult than Area 2. Many researchers have reported aphasic patients who could write only their name and/or other automatic written sequences (Ulatowska et al., 1979).

Category 2, comprised of Areas 4 and 5, focuses on the written production of single words. In Area 4 these are written in response to the spoken word, spoken letters, the printed word, or printed letters. In the latter two cases the printed forms are removed so that the patient has to rely to some extent on recall of the graphemic code. In Area 5, the aphasic patient is required to retrieve the lexical item (word) and then produce it graphemically, that is, written naming. Different varieties of cue support may be used to make this task easier (e.g., sentence completion). Therefore, Area 5 is more difficult than Area 4 for most patients.

Areas 6 and 7 compose Category 3, which requires semantic-syntactic linguistic processing for producing written grammatical structures. Therefore, patients who have problems with semantic word selection and forming grammatical units will require work in this category. This includes most aphasic patients, since their linguistic writing problems frequently parallel their oral expressive language problems. Area 7 represents an extension of Area 6 in requiring more complex material.

This current segmentation of areas represents two differences from those originally designed and used in the treatment data reported. These changes were motivated by the advances in recent views about writing. Area 4 has been expanded from spelling to dictation to include other input modalities. Area 6 has excluded the single-word level since this meshed better with the newly defined Areas 4 and 5. The reader will want to recall this when reading Chapters 12 and 13, which describe the treatment data.

Area 1: Tracing or Copying Nonverbal Material

Stimuli. Stimuli for this area focus on two- and three-dimensional representations of nonverbal material. These can range from simple geometric forms to more complicated designs and pictures of objects or actual objects. Subjects with apractic agraphia may also demonstrate constructional or drawing apraxia (Margolin and Binder, 1984) and be impaired in copying simple designs or geometric forms. When more complex designs (e.g., a cube rather than a square) are used, the aphasic subject also gets practice with appropriate spatial placement of forms or their component parts. Spatial aspects of graphic output are disturbed in subjects who show spatial agraphia.

Although there is no empirical evidence to develop a hierarchy among the stimuli, it seems clinically reasonable that simple designs will be easier than more complicated ones:

Geometric Forms:
    Three-dimensional
    Two-dimensional

Objects:
    Three-dimensional
    Two-dimensional

Geometric Designs

Description. The copying or tracing of materials is designed to activate or reactivate motor patterns of the arm and hand, which would correspond to the limb-motor graphic praxis.

Tracing objects and drawings is the basis of Visual Action Therapy (VAT) (Helm and Benson, 1978; Helm-Estabrooks et al., 1982). Step 1 of Level I involves having the global aphasic patient trace the examiner's hand and objects. Thus, VAT could be incorporated into LOT, first by using the graphic expression modality and later the gestural and gestural-verbal modality.

Example. The aphasic patient traces the line drawing of a knife.

Area 2: Tracing or Copying Verbal Material

1. Single Items

Stimuli. In aphasic subjects who demonstrate apraxic agraphia, the practic aspects of handwriting are impaired. Impairment in the store or organization of graphemic motor programs often results in unintelligible scrawl or scribbling, such that no graphemes can be identified. Since these subjects often show problems with incorrect letter elements, inappropriate spatial positioning, rotation of letters or elements, repetition of elements, and/or inappropriate orientation, tracing of letters and words are appropriate activities in treatment. When spatial agraphia accompanies the apractic agraphia, there may be problems with neglect of part of the writing space, irregular margins, repetitions of strokes or letters, and poor orientation of the lines of writing.

There has been no evidence that certain letters are more difficult than others, although individual patients will show different patterns. Stimuli include practice in graphically producing

Single letters
Single numbers
Single words

Description. Activities here are designed to activate or to enhance the graphemic motor patterns and/or spatial aspects necessary for producing handwriting. Some patients know the letter they want to write but they cannot activate or produce the appropriate graphemic motor patterns. In some patients both tracing and copying will be used; in others, only copying may be required. The outcome of these activities is to have the patient produce legible graphemes rather than a scrawl.

Example. The aphasic patient copies single letters.

2. Items in a Series

Stimuli. The stimuli are the same as those listed for single items, except that they are now presented in series. Again, there are no empirical data for arranging them in a hierarchy:

Series of letters
Series of numbers
Series of words

Description. These activities require the aphasic patient to attend to and persist with more extended series.

Example. The aphasic patient copies the number series that corresponds to his or her telephone number.

Area 3: Writing Familiar Material

Responses. The aphasic patient is required to recall the graphemic elements and the corresponding motor patterns for highly overlearned material. There is no hierarchy established, with the exception that the patient's name is probably the easiest:

Name
Age
Address
Alphabet
Numbers in sequential order
   (e.g., 1 to 20)

Description. These activities are designed to aid the aphasic individual in recalling and producing very familiar, highly overlearned material.

Example. The aphasic patient is given a blank check and asked to write his or her name. The appropriate space is indicated with an X.

Area 4: Written Spelling

Stimuli. There are several ways that stimuli can be presented to the aphasic patient for written spelling. When presented auditorily, the patient hears the entire word and writes it. If the word is spelled, the patient has only to write the graphemic counterpart of a series of letter names. Some aphasic patients are able to perform this task but have difficulty segmenting a word into its component sounds and are, consequently, unable to write a dictated sound (e.g., /b/) rather than a letter name (e.g., /bi/) for "b" (Shallice, 1981). Words can also be shown visually and then removed, either in their entirety or with sequentially presented letters. No available data show significant differences among these presentation methods for these stimuli:

Auditory word
Orally spelled word
Printed word
Printed letter series

Whether requested to respond by writing in cursive or manuscript did not seem to influence the accuracy of writing in a group of aphasic patients. Since individual subjects differed considerably in their success using one form versus the other, Boone and Friedman (1976) recommended that the individual's preference and best performance form be used in treatment. Consistent with performance in other language modalities, length and frequency of occurrence of the stimulus words affect performance. Aphasic subjects generally spell high frequency words more accurately than low frequency words (Beauvois and Dérouesné, 1981; Bricker, Schuell, and Jenkins, 1964; Langmore and Canter, 1983). In general, longer words occasion more errors than shorter ones (Beauvois and Dérouesné, 1981; Bricker et al., 1964; Langmore and Canter, 1983; Roeltgen et al., 1983). Most errors tended to occur in the middle of words rather than at the end, regardless of the word length, suggesting that memory was not the factor responsible for the length effect (Roeltgen et al., 1983). Langmore and Canter (1983) reported that there was a disproportionate increase in the number of errors for long words than would be predicted simply by the increase in the number of letters. This information has been incorporated into two hierarchies, which list stimuli from easy to difficult.

Easy ↓ Difficult	High frequency words
	Low frequency words

Easy	Short words
	Long words
	Increase in letters
↓ Difficult	Increase in syllables

The degree of orthography, or how closely the sound of a word corresponds to its spelling, significantly influences some aphasic patients, those who demonstrate lexical dysgraphia (Beauvois and Dérouesné, 1981; Roeltgen and Heilman, 1984). One study that used groups of aphasic patients also found this effect, at least in some patients (Wapner and Gardner, 1979). The hierarchy listed below lists findings from easiest to most difficult; however, some of the differences between word groups were not statistically significant.

Easy ↓ Difficult	Anterior Patients	Posterior Patients
	Words with double vowel	Words with regular spelling
	Words with double consonant	Words with double vowel
	Words with homonyms	Words with double consonant
	Words with regular spelling	Words with silent letters
	Words with silent letters	Words with homonyms

The ambiguity of words, that is, whether they can be spelled in only one way (e.g., charm) or whether they can be spelled with more than one graphemic sequence (e.g., cotton, kotton, or cotten) also affects spelling performance in lexical agraphic individuals. Aphasic patients made fewer spelling errors on low ambiguity words written to dictation (Beauvois and Dérouesné, 1981; Roeltgen and Heilman, 1984).

Words with homonyms (words that sound alike but are spelled differently) were among the harder words for the aphasic subjects studied by Wapner and Gardner (1979). Roeltgen and colleagues (1982) found that their aphasic patients with lexical agraphia could spell the homonyms correctly but frequently selected the wrong one to fit the linguistic context (e.g., The *sale* on the boat ripped).

The phonetic and morphological character of words influenced the patients with Broca's aphasia in Langmore and Canter's study (1983). They made more errors on consonants than vowels and more errors on words that contained suffixes than those that did not. The hierarchies for these variables, from easy to difficult, follow.

Easy	Consonants
↓	
Difficult	Vowels

Easy	Nonsuffixed words
↓	
Difficult	Suffixed words

Other factors important to spelling performance are (1) imageability: high imageable (e.g., *book*) or low imageable (e.g., *law*) words; (2) concreteness: concrete (e.g., *hat*) or abstract (e.g., *hope*) words; and (3) grammatical class (e.g., nouns, verbs, adjectives, function words). The deep agraphic patient described by Bub and Kertesz (1982a), the four phonological agraphic cases described by Roeltgen and co-workers (1983), and the agrammatic patients of Martin, Caramazza, and Berndt (1982) showed effects of one or more of these variables. The concrete-abstract and imageability variables, although not synonymous, would be highly correlated. Therefore, the results have been pooled here for the hierarchy, listing from easiest to most difficult. When two items appear on the same line, they were considered to be of equivalent difficulty. The verb category was listed twice because in one study it appeared equivalent to low imagery nouns and to function words in another.

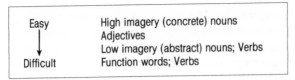

Easy	High imagery (concrete) nouns
↓	Adjectives
	Low imagery (abstract) nouns; Verbs
Difficult	Function words; Verbs

Whether a letter sequence forms a word or not influences the performance of individuals who demonstrate phonological agraphia. In these patients the phoneme-grapheme conversion route to spelling is damaged. Since nonwords or pseudowords are not represented in the lexicon because they have no meaning, they must be spelled via the phonological route. Although Bub and Kertesz (1982b) found a slight difference between mono- and polysyllabic nonwords, others have not commented on the effect of length.

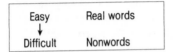

Easy	Real words
↓	
Difficult	Nonwords

Roeltgen and associates (1983) examined the effect of emotionality, defined by the examiners subjectively as emotional or neutral, on written spelling in three subjects with phonological agraphia. For one subject, there was no difference in performance between emotional and neutral words. Since two patients did show effects a tentative hierarchy is listed. These results need to be replicated before firm conclusions can be drawn. The list is ranked from easiest to most difficult.

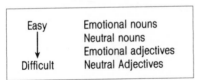

Easy	Emotional nouns
↓	Neutral nouns
	Emotional adjectives
Difficult	Neutral Adjectives

Description. Activities here are designed to have the aphasic patient produce correct written spelling. The wide variety of variables affecting performance on these tasks has been described above.

Example. The clinician presents a series of concrete, high frequency, monosyllabic words to an aphasic patient for writing. The words are functional for hospital needs (e.g., *bed, food, television*).

Area 5: Written Naming

Written naming is somewhat similar to spelling in that the aphasic patient is required to write a word. In this case, however, there is the added step of having to select the appropriate word and then spell it correctly. This area of written naming concentrates on the word selection process rather than the spelling. Understandably, the same factors will affect performance as listed in Area 4 if spelling is the major difficulty.

Stimuli. The stimuli for written naming tasks are frequently objects or pictures presented by the examiner; these have come to be known as confrontation naming tasks. Bub and Kertesz (1982b) found slightly better performance with objects as stimuli compared with pictures.

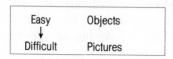

The effect of the length of a word was investigated by Friederici and co-workers (1981) for Broca's and Wernicke's aphasic patients. The effect of length was very striking, with short single-syllable words easier than three-syllable words.

The fewest errors occurred in the middle of the words, followed by the end of the word, and then the beginning. The hierarchies from easiest to most difficult are outlined below.

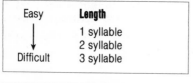

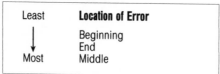

The lack of a significant overall frequency effect could be explained by the small difference between the high and low frequency words (25 versus 15 occurrences per million). However, there was a significant interaction between frequency of occurrence and degree of phoneme-grapheme correspondence. If the spelling of a word utilized the most regular expression of phoneme-grapheme correspondence (P-G) rules, it was termed high frequency P-G (e.g., /ʃ/ in *ship*). Low frequency P-G rules were those in which the letter combination in the spelling was a less frequent realization of the sounds (e.g., /f/ in rou*gh*). The following hierarchy from most to least correct is reproduced from Friederici and colleagues (1981).

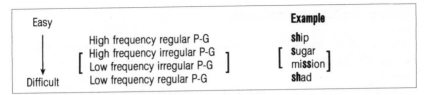

Response. Although written naming tasks are included in aphasia test batteries, the stimulus range evaluated is small. Most of the work in the area has been concerned with the type of errors patients made rather than with the stimuli used to elicit them. Therefore, some attention has been given to responses. An attempt has been made to dissociate naming and spelling errors and an adapted response hierarchy from Schuell and Jenkins (1961) is proposed.

Responses	Example
Correct	house
Approximate	hows
Target word is recognizable but spelled incorrectly	
Semantically associated	porch
Associated with the target word in some meaningful manner	
No response or no appropriate response	banana

Correct responses require selection of the appropriate word and its correct spelling. Approximate responses, as recognizable attempts at the target, suggest that the patient has selected the appropriate word but has misspelled it. (The type of spelling error can be analyzed for whether the phonological or lexical route appears to be used by a particular patient.) Semantically associated responses include responses that bear a semantic relation to the target word. They might be an in-class substitution (e.g., fork/spoon), a functional association (e.g., pour/pitcher), a meaningful relationship (e.g., time/clock), and so forth. Semantic errors, depending on their degree of association to the target, would not necessarily allow the listener to identify the specific target word but would provide more or less information about the topic. No response or no appropriate response gives the listener no relevant information about the target word. The response might be a real word, a neologism, or illegible (e.g., motorcycle/towel rack; /klɪ pɔ˞mɛk/ for book).

Description. Activities in written naming reflect another approach to word retrieval problems. The aphasic person is asked to produce in written form the name of an object, action, and so on. For some aphasic patients, such as some Broca's, written naming is superior to oral naming.

Example. The clinician presents a picture of an action (e.g., walk) and the aphasic patient writes the corresponding action word.

Area 6: Written Formulation

In written formulation the aphasic patient formulates grammatical structures rather than single words. These may be produced in response to a picture or object presented by the clinician. Alternatively, the clinician may suggest a topic, such as an event experienced by the patient, or request the written recall of a paragraph read to the patient.

Responses. Written formulation responses vary in their length and complexity. Most of the literature has described aphasic patients' responses using rather open-ended tasks. Therefore, evidence is sparse regarding how to directly affect these aspects. Because aphasic patients' writing is reduced in quantity and often limited in length and presence or variety of grammatical structures, these appeared to be relevant variables to control. The guidelines from oral formulation might be of assistance here, since the linguistic deficits in speaking and writing parallel one another to some extent (Goodglass and Hunter, 1970; Ulatowska et al., 1979; Weisenburg and McBride, 1935).

1. Phrases
    High Familiarity   **Example**
    Short   cup of soup
    Long   cup of tomato soup
    Low Familiarity
    Short   Boston ivy
    Long   trailing Boston ivy
2. Sentences
    High Familiarity
    Short   I'm fine.
    Long   I can hear you now.
    Low Familiarity
    Short   The spice spilled.
    Long   The painter put more oil in the
                                                        furnace.

3. Paragraphs
    High Familiarity
    Short   2 sentences; 3 to 5 words;
                                                        topic: family

    Long   4 sentences; 5 to 7 words;
                                                        topic: family

    Low Familiarity
    Short   2 sentences; 3 to 5 words;
                                                        topic: a picnic

    Long   4 sentences; 5 to 7 words;
                                                        topic: a picnic

Grammatical complexity is generally simple in aphasic individual's writing. Ulatowska and co-workers (1979) found that most sentences were simple and affirmative. Aphasic patients in treatment produced a high number of compound sentences but few complex ones.

Sentence Type	Example
Simple	
NP + V + NP	The boy has a cookie.
NP + V	The girl is dancing.
NP + be + COMP	The wagon is red.
NP + V + ADV	The man walks slowly.
Compound	She is washing, and the kids are playing.
Complex	She is crying because the dog is lost.

Ulatowska and co-workers (1979) used the measure of clause per sentence ratio for complexity of narrative paragraph production in response to the "Cookie Theft" picture.

Clausal elements can also be analyzed in written performance. The little data that are available stem from the observations of Ulatowska and colleagues (1979). The suggestions below come from this work.

Noun Phrase Elements	Example
Noun	boy
Modifier + Noun	big boy
$\left[\begin{array}{c} \text{Article}^1 \\ \text{Possessive} \end{array} \right]$ + (Quantifier) + (Adjective) + Noun	the big boy
	her big boy

Omission of definite and indefinite articles were the most frequent errors for this category. Prepositional phrases can be expanded in a similar manner to noun phrases. Omission of the preposition was the most frequent error found.

Verb Forms	Example
Simple present	I eat.
Present progressive	I am eating.
Simple past	I ate.
Modals	
Marking future	I will eat.
Marking intention or ability	I can eat.
Auxiliaries	
Be, have	I have eaten.
	I had eaten.
	I have been eating.

The most frequent verb errors were omission of the auxiliary in the present progressive, followed by a shift from past to present tense.

---

[1] Only one item within the braces can be selected. The items in brackets can be selected optionally to expand the noun phrase.

Another aspect that must be woven into treatment in this area is increasing the amount of content in the writing of those aphasic patients who tend to write using nonspecific terms, such as "thing," "it," "around," and so on. This is most commonly found in Wernicke's aphasic patients.

Punctuation is frequently omitted by aphasic subjects, and capitalization is often incorrect. A grammar book used in the school system can be of help in organizing these aspects of writing with those aphasic patients for whom it is appropriate.

With paragraph writing, the elements of discourse are added to the writing task. When producing a narrative, certain aspects of discourse are obligatory and others are optional. To some extent, whether the optional ones are used depends on the stimulus material. The system here is from Labov (cited in Freedman-Stern et al., 1984):

Inclusion		Structure of Discourse
Optional	1.	Abstract: a statement about the content of the narrative
Most contain it	2.	Orientation: information about the setting (time and place) and identification of the participants (actors)
Obligatory	3.	Complicating action: a series of clauses that relate the event
Probably necessary	4.	Evaluation: indication(s) of how the speaker feels about the event
Most contain it	5.	Result or resolution: a statement of the final event(s)
Optional	6.	Coda: the moral of the story

Writing a paragraph requires the inclusion of a complicating action and most probably an orientation and a result. In addition, the clausal units must be linked cohesively with mechanisms such as dependent relative, temporal, or causative (finite and nonfinite) clauses or independent clauses conjoined with "but." In addition, pronouns serve as a cohesive device when used anaphorically (for example, The *boy* ate the fish. *He* was full. *He* is used to refer to a previously specified noun [*boy*].) Deictic reference (here, there, this, that) is another way of creating cohesion in written discourse (e.g., *This* lamp goes *here* in the corner; *that one* goes beside the table). Work on written discourse in the aphasia literature is limited to the studies of Ulatowska and colleagues (1979) and Freedman-Stern and associates (1984). Most of these data dealt with discourse longer than a paragraph and will be described in Area 7 to come. It is important to note that the older normal subjects studied did not use a narrative style in the picture description task although almost 25 percent of the aphasic subjects did and achieved cohesion through a variety of devices. Ulatowska and co-workers (1979) noted that although grammatical structure at the sentence level was disturbed, the structure of discourse was preserved. The following are suggestions for discourse at the paragraph level in work with aphasic patients. The clincian starts with the obligatory elements and adds other elements until a complete narrative is produced.

Obligatory Elements of Narrative

Complication action
Orientation or result
Orientation and result
Evaluation
Abstract or coda
Abstract and coda

Cohesive Devices

Select appropriate items and increase their number and variety
Anaphoric reference
Deixis
Relative clauses
Temporal ordering
Causative clauses
Conditional clauses

Description. Activities in this area are designed to improve the patient's ability to use written language as a mode of communication. The activities increase in difficulty along several parameters: length, grammatical complexity, semantic content, cohesion, and discourse. Attention is also given to punctuation as it becomes appropriate.

Example. The aphasic person is asked to write a simple sentence about his or her occupation.

Area 7: Writing Complex Material

Area 7 is meant to represent a more complex level of Area 6. At this level, the patient extends beyond a single paragraph and the typical tasks of describing his or her job or a picture presented.

Responses. The responses to come all involve one form of discourse or another. They conceivably vary in their familiarity to the patient and also in their length. Type of discourse aside, shorter and more familiar topics will probably be easier for the patient. The single patient described by Freedman-Stern and colleagues (1984) showed the following discourse hierarchy from easiest to most difficult. Whether other patients will show a similar rank order remains to be tested.

| Narrative: | language representation of an event or series of events in which a sequence of clauses is matched to the sequence of events | **Example** "My Summer Vacation" |

| Letter: | conventional structure: greeting, conventional opening (or statement of purpose in a formal letter), body (variable, may contain an embedded narrative), conventional closing, and salutation | Letter to a relative |
| Expository: | subject matter–oriented discourse organized by logical linkages | Growing roses |

Types of complex material that could be classified into various types of discourse are

Essay
Short story
Business report
Newspaper column

Variables to consider controlling are the same as those for discourse discussed in Area 6.

Structure of discourse
Length
Complexity of grammatical structures
Cohesion devices

Cohesive devices were an important variable in the effectiveness of written discourse (Freedman-Stern et al., 1984) and syntactic complexity appeared to be related to cohesion. If the cohesive linkages could be expressed with simple grammatical devices, this led to more effective discourse. Problems in using complex syntactic forms, therefore, may have prevented achieving coherence that, in turn, led to a less effective text.

Description. Activities in this area are of a high level of difficulty. They require the aphasic patient to express thoughts in some logical order, to produce grammatically correct sentences, to spell and punctuate correctly, and to provide information to the reader. These activities are generally appropriate for patients for whom writing was premorbidly important, especially those for whom it is important in a job or career. They are also appropriate for the rare patient whose writing is better than other modalities and for whom written communication is the modality of choice.

Example. The aphasic patient, a former newspaper columnist, is asked to write a newspaper article reporting a football game seen on television.

Chapter 11

Materials for Graphic Expression

Area 1: Tracing and Copying Nonverbal Material

Beginning Levels

Level 1

Stimuli. Two-dimensional drawings of functionally familiar objects

Set A		Set B	
1.	cup	1.	toothbrush
2.	paintbrush	2.	spoon
3.	tree	3.	razor
4.	knife	4.	pot
5.	pipe	5.	door
6.	saw	6.	ladder
7.	hat	7.	shoe
8.	chair	8.	bed
9.	comb	9.	fork
10.	hammer	10.	bowl

Procedure. The clinician presents a drawing and the patient is required to trace it.

Level 2

Stimuli. Two-dimensional drawings of objects

Set A		Set B	
1.	cup	1.	toothbrush
2.	paintbrush	2.	spoon
3.	tree	3.	razor
4.	knife	4.	pot
5.	pipe	5.	door
6.	saw	6.	ladder
7.	hat	7.	lollipop
8.	chair	8.	bed
9.	comb	9.	fork
10.	hammer	10.	bowl

Procedure. The clinician presents a line drawing and the patient is required to copy it.

Level 3

Stimuli. Two-dimensional drawings of objects

Set A		Set B	
1.	cup	1.	toothbrush
2.	paintbrush	2.	spoon
3.	tree	3.	razor
4.	knife	4.	pot
5.	pipe	5.	door
6.	saw	6.	ladder
7.	hat	7.	lollipop
8.	chair	8.	bed
9.	comb	9.	fork
10.	hammer	10.	bowl

Procedure. The clinician presents a line drawing for 10 seconds, and the patient is required to draw it from memory.

Additional Levels

Additional levels may be developed by introducing more complex line drawings and by adding a third dimension.

Area 2: Tracing and Copying Verbal Material

1. Single Items

Beginning Levels

Level 1

Stimuli. Printed or cursive single letters

Set A	Set B
1. E	1. S
2. O	2. U
3. A	3. X
4. D	4. B
5. Z	5. H
6. R	6. L
7. F	7. W
8. I	8. T
9. D	9. C
10. G	10. M

Procedure. The clinician presents a printed letter, and the patient is required to copy it.

Level 2

Stimuli. Single numbers

Set A

1. 8
2. 2
3. 3
4. 7
5. 1
6. 9
7. 4
8. 0
9. 6
10. 5

Procedure. The clinician presents a number, and the patient is required to copy it.

Level 3

Stimuli. Printed single words; three letters long, grades 1 to 4 vocabulary

Set A	Set B
1. FOR	1. CAR
2. DAY	2. GET
3. SUN	3. YES
4. NOT	4. NOW
5. BOX	5. TRY
6. CUP	6. MEN

7.	ANY	7.	SIX
8.	LIP	8.	HOT
9.	WHO	9.	WAR
10.	RAN	10.	JOB

Procedure. The clinician presents a word, and the patient is required to copy it.

Single Items: Additional Levels

Additional levels could be formed by increasing the length of numbers and words.

2. Items in a Series

Beginning Levels

Level 1

Stimuli. Printed series of words

Set A		Set B	
1.	R I A D	1.	A K O H
2.	O P Q F	2.	D E V C
3.	C L V N	3.	P I M G
4.	T I B Z	4.	F Q Y U
5.	U E H M	5.	Z H N J
6.	X W J G	6.	B G K T
7.	Y P N C	7.	J X D M
8.	K A S F	8.	N A B L
9.	D O B T	9.	C R I E
10.	T Z P I	10.	S L F W

Procedure. The clinician presents a series of printed letters, and the patient is required to copy it.

Level 2

Stimuli. Series of numbers

Set A		Set B	
1.	693–0712	1.	590–6832
2.	584–6972	2.	764–9206
3.	310–2350	3.	471–5639
4.	921–5460	4.	679–0215
5.	203–1892	5.	375–9876
6.	754–3681	6.	201–3547

7.	415–7069	7.	897–6431
8.	834–5176	8.	971–2865
9.	915–2376	9.	453–8967
10.	834–5210	10.	375–6248

Procedure. The clinician presents a series of numbers, and the patient is required to copy it.

Level 3

Stimuli. Printed series of words

Set A

1.	PAY	LIP	GOT
2.	DOG	CAN	FLY
3.	TIE	EGG	SUN
4.	BED	THE	ICE
5.	ATE	GEM	LAP
6.	CRY	OWN	INK
7.	HAT	FEE	BUY
8.	RED	SEA	PIG
9.	ONE	FAR	JET
10.	MEN	EEL	APE

Set B

1.	TOP	BAD	OFF
2.	DUE	CAR	SAW
3.	ADD	RUN	ZOO
4.	CUP	TRY	FOE
5.	WHY	KEG	EAR
6.	PIE	BUD	HOE
7.	SIT	AGO	DEN
8.	TWO	DAM	BEE
9.	LAP	NET	MOM
10.	BIG	SAY	PUT

Procedure. The clinician presents a printed series of words, and the patient is required to copy it.

Items in a Series: Additional Levels

Additional levels may be developed by increasing the length and number of words in the series.

Area 3: Writing Familiar Material

Beginning Levels

Level 1

Stimuli. Printed segments of highly familiar material, with one element omitted

Set A

1.	Wednesday	Thursday	_____	Saturday
2.	One	two	_____	four
3.	D	____	F	G
4.	January	February	March	_____

5. 6   7   ____   9
6. H   ____   J   K
7. ____   12   13   14
8. _____   July   August   September
9. Monday   Tuesday   Wednesday   _____
10. W   X   ____   Z

Set B

1. L   M   N   ____
2. thirty-one   _____   thirty-three   thirty-four
3. Friday   Saturday   _____   Monday
4. A   B   ____   D
5. _____   October   November   December
6. 17   18   19   ____
7. Q   ____   S   T
8. _____   May   June   July
9. U   V   W   ____
10. 72   73   ____   75

Procedure. The segments of printed words are presented, and the patient is required to write in the missing element.

Level 2

Stimuli. Highly overlearned material

Set A

1. name
2. address
3. letters of the alphabet

Set B

1. numbers from 1 to 20
2. days of the week
3. months of the year

Procedure. The clinician requests the patient to write the elements of a given series.

Level 3

Stimuli. Blank check; body of a letter

Procedure

Set A

The patient is provided with a blank check and is required to fill in the date, the name of a family member, an amount of money, and the signature.

Set B

The patient is provided with the body of a letter and is required to fill in the address, the date, the salutation, and the signature.

Area 4: Written Spelling

The following material was designed for patients demonstrating pure alexia.

Beginning Levels

Level 1

Stimuli. Nouns, three letters in length; grades 1 to 4 vocabulary

Set A		Set B	
1.	bag	1.	car
2.	saw	2.	hat
3.	leg	3.	box
4.	pan	4.	cat
5.	dog	5.	van
6.	fan	6.	sun
7.	jar	7.	rug
8.	gun	8.	boy
9.	cup	9.	net
10.	bee	10.	cow

Procedure. The clinician orally provides a word, and the patient is required to write it.

Level 2

Stimuli. Nouns, five letters in length; grades 1 to 4 vocabulary

Set A		Set B	
1.	paper	1.	water
2.	woman	2.	peach
3.	motor	3.	motel
4.	teeth	4.	tiger
5.	cabin	5.	honey
6.	juice	6.	canoe
7.	piano	7.	money
8.	robin	8.	lemon
9.	queen	9.	mouse
10.	salad	10.	sugar

Procedures. The clinician orally provides a word, and the patient is required to write it.

Level 3

Stimuli. Nouns, 8 to 10 letters in length; grades 1 to 4 vocabulary

Set A	Set B
1. president	1. business
2. something	2. department
3. mountain	3. territory
4. permission	4. condition
5. telephone	5. moonlight
6. difficulty	6. fountain
7. candidate	7. necessity
8. building	8. humanity
9. governor	9. suffering
10. ceremony	10. machinery

Procedure. The clinician orally provides a word, and the patient is requested to write it.

Additional Levels

Additional levels may be developed by increasing the grade level of vocabulary and the word length and by incorporating verbs, adjectives, and functor words.

Area 5: Written Naming

Beginning Levels

Level 1

Stimuli. Pictured nouns, one syllable and four letters in length; regular grapheme-phoneme correspondence; grades 1 to 4 vocabulary

Set A	Set B
1. bird	1. moon
2. coat	2. game
3. lake	3. feet
4. salt	4. cape
5. nose	5. shoe
6. meat	6. neck
7. robe	7. wall
8. hair	8. bank
9. gift	9. star
10. wine	10. pope

Procedure. A pictured noun is placed in front of the patient, who is required to write its name.

Level 2

Stimuli. Pictured nouns, two syllables and six letters in length; regular phoneme-grapheme correspondence; grades 1 to 4 vocabulary

Set A   **Set B**

	Set A		Set B
1.	hammer	1.	rabbit
2.	pocket	2.	number
3.	finger	3.	letter
4.	tunnel	4.	dinner
5.	butter	5.	garden
6.	window	6.	carpet
7.	ribbon	7.	ticket
8.	dragon	8.	flower
9.	basket	9.	record
10.	fabric	10.	helmet

Procedure. A pictured noun is placed in front of the patient, who is required to write its name.

Level 3

Stimuli. Pictured nouns, one syllable and four to six letters in length; irregular phoneme-grapheme correspondence; grades 1 to 4 vocabulary

Set A   **Set B**

	Set A		Set B
1.	knee	1.	town
2.	light	2.	glove
3.	ghost	3.	fence
4.	flood	4.	noise
5.	sauce	5.	thread
6.	tomb	6.	knife
7.	thumb	7.	lamb
8.	monk	8.	wound
9.	reign	9.	worm
10.	breast	10.	bough

Procedure. A pictured noun is placed in front of the patient, who is required to write its name.

Additional Levels

Additional levels may be developed by increasing the grade level of vocabulary and the word length and by incorporating verbs, adjectives, and functor words.

Area 6: Written Formulation

Beginning Levels

Level 1

Stimuli. Pictured nouns to elicit highly familiar phrases; two to four syllables in length; grades 1 to 4 vocabulary

Set A   Set B

1.	deep water	1.	white dress
2.	big house	2.	sweet fruit
3.	black cat	3.	little chair
4.	bright light	4.	pretty girl
5.	busy cook	5.	wild flowers
6.	fat woman	6.	straight hair
7.	soft pillow	7.	polite boy
8.	old woman	8.	tight pants
9.	clean hands	9.	funny face
10.	sick child	10.	dirty shirt

Procedure. A picture corresponding to a two-word phrase is presented. The patient is required to write the phrase.

Level 2

Stimuli. Action pictures to elicit highly familiar sentences; seven to nine syllables in length; grades 1 to 4 vocabulary; NP + V + NP construction; present progressive verb tense

Procedure. An action picture is placed in front of the patient, who is required to write a short sentence describing the activity.

Set A

1. The man is washing the car.
2. The child is sleeping in the bed.
3. The boy is eating his lunch.
4. The dog is burying a bone.
5. The teacher is writing on the board.
6. The woman is making the bed.
7. The baby is throwing the ball.
8. The people are singing a song.
9. The farmer is driving a truck.
10. The cook is making breakfast.

Set B

1. The mother is walking in the park.
2. The girl is drinking her milk.
3. The cat is sitting on the table.
4. The children are running a race.
5. The bird is building a nest.
6. The women are playing cards.
7. The tailor is sewing the pants.
8. The artist is painting a picture.
9. The robber is taking the jewels.
10. The clerk is selling a shirt.

Level 3

Stimuli. Sets of two simple sentences to be combined to form one complex sentence, 13 to 16 syllables in length; grades 1 to 4 vocabulary; present tense

Set A

1. a. The doctor is driving to the hospital.
    b. The doctor is nervous.
    Response: The doctor who is nervous is driving to the hospital.
2. a. The victim is telling her story.
    b. The story is dreadful.
    Response: The victim is telling a story that is dreadful.
3. a. The gallery is remarkable.
    b. It has a new director.
    Response: The gallery that has a new director is remarkable.
4. a. The traveler is visiting France.
    b. The traveler is a teacher.
    Response: The traveler who is a teacher is visiting France.
5. a. The policeman is chasing the robber.
    b. The robber is violent.
    Response: The policeman is chasing the robber who is violent.
6. a. The woman is stopping traffic.
    b. The woman is desperate.
    Response: The woman who is desperate is stopping traffic.
7. a. The farmer sells his vegetables.
    b. The vegetables are always fresh.
    Response: The farmer sells his vegetables, which are always fresh.
8. a. His beautiful daughter curls her hair.
    b. Her hair is very straight.
    Response: His beautiful daughter curls her hair, which is very
        straight.

9. a. My mother often reads novels.
   b. The novels are unusual.
   Response: My mother often reads novels that are unusual.
10. a. The cabinet stands in the parlor.
    b. The cabinet is broken.
    Response: The cabinet that is broken stands in the parlor.

Set B

1. a. The cook is organizing dinner.
   b. He is in the kitchen.
   Response: The cook who is organizing dinner is in the kitchen.
2. a. The child plays the piano.
   b. He practices every day.
   Response. The child who plays the piano practices every day.
3. a. The large box is on the table.
   b. It contains old clothes.
   Response: The large box that is on the table contains old clothes.
4. a. The man is working in the garden.
   b. He is retired.
   Response: The man is who is working in the garden is retired.
5. a. The couple is going to the cabin.
   b. The cabin is on the lake.
   Response: The couple is going to the cabin that is on the lake.
6. a. The boy is painting the ceiling.
   b. He is a painter.
   Response: The boy who is painting the ceiling is a painter.
7. a. The children listen to music.
   b. The music is usually loud.
   Response: The children listen to music that is usually loud.
8. a. The butcher prepared the meat.
   b. The meat is expensive.
   Response: The butcher prepared the meat, which is expensive.
9. a. The building is very bright.
   b. It has many windows.
   Response: The building that has many windows is very bright.
10. a. His dad is furnishing the house.
    b. The house is in the country.
    Response: His dad is furnishing the house, which is in the country.

Procedure. Two sentences are presented orally to the patient, who is required to combine them into one complex written sentence. The sentences could also be presented in written form.

Additional Levels

Additional levels may be developed by increasing the length and grammatical complexity of the output. Use of punctuation and capitalization may also be incorporated.

Area 7: Writing Complex Material

Beginning Levels

Level 1

Procedure. The patient is required to write a narrative about (1) a television program recently viewed and (2) a newspaper article recently read.

Level 2

Procedure. The patient is required to write (1) a letter to a friend and (2) a letter to a company regarding poor delivery service.

Level 3

Procedure. The patient is required to write an expository paragraph describing (1) organizing a wedding and (2) buying a new house.

Additional Levels

Additional levels may be developed by increasing the length and complexity of the output required.

Chapter 12

Subjects, Procedures, and Efficacy Data for the LOT Study

As part of a large study on language therapy and recovery from aphasia (Shewan and Kertesz, 1984), LOT was one type of treatment used with a group of patients. This chapter will describe the characteristics of this group and the tests and procedures used to study them. The LOT group did not differ significantly from any of the other treatment groups included in the larger study for variables of age, education, socioeconomic status, type, and severity. This suggested that the LOT group to be described was representative of the more general aphasic population studied.

A second purpose of this chapter is to present data demonstrating that LOT is an efficacious type of treatment. Language treatment has been provided by speech-language pathologists for aphasic patients for several decades. Most treatment methods used have not been subjected to studies of their efficacy. Of the few investigations that have demonstrated the efficacy of language treatment, therapy methods employed have not been described in sufficient detail to allow for replication by clinicians in the field. Now that LOT has been described in detail in the preceding chapters, the data demonstrating its efficacy will be presented.

SUBJECTS

The subjects who received LOT came from the larger patient group referred to the Language Therapy and Recovery from Aphasia Project

(Shewan and Kertesz, 1983). Over the course of almost 3 years of data collection, 281 subjects were referred to the project by neurologists and family physicians. Patients came from London and the surrounding region of southwestern Ontario.

The referral pattern of subjects was examined on a month-to-month basis and in 6-month time intervals. The number of referrals varied from a low of 1 to a high of 23. In general, the number of patients who met the entry criteria and who were, therefore, accepted into the study was directly related to the total referral pattern ($r = 0.823$). Each year was divided into 6-month time spans (Winter = October to March, Summer = April to September) to determine if there was any recurring referral pattern related to time of year. The cold winter climate and its snow shoveling might have influenced the incidence of stroke seasonally. Data were collected over six times spans, with the last one representing a 4-month rather than a 6-month period. Table 12–1 shows the referral and acceptance pattern across this time span. The total number of referrals varied from 29 to 107 per 6-month period. However, there was no significant difference between the mean number of referrals for the Winter and Summer periods ($p > .05$). Although there were no significant seasonal differences, the trend appeared to be a decline in the number of referrals across time. This could have reflected a declining interest in the study by referring physicians as time passed. However, with frequent reminders for referrals and the high visibility of the study, this did not appear to be the most plausible explanation. Alternatively, physicians may have become more familiar with the entry criteria for the study and, at later stages, did not refer patients who were inappropriate. This would have the effect of decreasing the total number of referrals. In addition, advances in stroke prevention may have influenced the incidence figures and, consequently, the referral pattern. Aspirin has been shown to reduce the incidence of stroke in the male population (The Canadian Co-operative Study Group, 1978) treated for transient ischemic attacks (TIAs). Since London was a major centre in this study and since this was a current method of treatment during data collection and is currently, at least by some physicians, this could reduce the number of stroke patients (and aphasic patients) in the area. Another major London research project was investigating the management of hypertension (Bass, Donner, and McWhinney, 1982). Since hypertension is a highly frequent risk factor for stroke, controlling hypertension may be gradually reducing the number of strokes. Additionally, there is increasing public awareness of the risk factors for stroke, and people may be seeking medical attention in the preventable stages. Therefore, earlier detection of the risk of stroke (TIA, hypertension, and so on) and early treatment (aspirin, hypertension control) may be operating to reduce the incidence.

Table 12-1. Referral and Acceptance Pattern of Subjects Across Data Collection Period

Time Period	Number of Referrals	Number of Acceptances	Percent Acceptance
1978			
Summer	29	8	27.6
1979			
Winter	107	39	36.4
Summer	81	34	42.0
1980			
Winter	33	14	42.4
Summer	50	20	40.0
1981			
Winter*	34.5	19.5	56.5

*Data collection period was 4 months only. The values presented were prorated to represent a 6-month period.

The percentage of accepted patients, compared with the total referrals, gradually increased throughout the data collection period. This may have also reflected physicians' increasing familiarity with the entry criteria for the study. As time passed and they had reviewed the criteria more frequently, they may have tended to exclude patients who did not meet the criteria, for example, patients who had had a previous stroke. If this were the case, both fewer referrals and a higher percentage of referrals meeting the entry criteria would be expected. This was the pattern observed.

Of the referral group, 100 subjects met the entry criteria outlined in Table 12–2. The age cutoffs of 18 years and 85 years were used so as to include only adult subjects, defined as 18 years or older, who had a reasonable probability of being able to participate in the study for one year. Extending the age range beyond 85 was decided against because of the high mortality rate in this age group in the normal population without stroke.

Education was not strictly controlled as an entry criterion. However, because the test battery included reading and writing components and because aphasia affects the reading and writing modalities, only subjects who were literate were included. Literacy was determined in an interview with the family of the aphasic subject.

The course of recovery from aphasia in different etiological groups has sometimes been reported to be different. For example, Eisenson (1984) and Butfield and Zangwill (1946) reported better recovery in aphasic patients of traumatic etiology than of cerebrovascular origin. By contrast, Gloning, Trappl, Heiss, and Quatember (1976) did not find etiology to be a

Table 12–2.   Entry and Exit Criteria for Aphasic Subjects

Criterion Variable	
	ENTRY CRITERIA
Age	18 to 85 yr
Education	Literacy by history

Etiology	Infarcts
	Stable intracerebral hemorrhages
	Excluded hemorrhages due to
	    AV malformation
	    Subarachnoid hemorrhage
	    Aneurysm
	Single unilateral strokes
	TIAs (5 days or less) excluded

Medical status	Excluded unstable medical illnesses interfering with testing or survival
Sensory status	Passed hearing screening for age appropriateness Blind patients (defined clinically) excluded Tactile dysfunction not excluded
Time post onset	2 to 4 weeks post stroke
Language severity	Native speakers of English or competent bilinguals for whom treatment in English was appropriate Severe language barrier or accent excluded
	EXIT CRITERIA
Language recovery	WAB LQ of 94.0 or above
Death	Subject died
Second stroke	Neurological deficit persisting longer than 5 days
Prolonged illness	Absense or illness longer than 3 weeks' duration
Geographical relocation	Subject moved
Voluntary withdrawal	Subject did not wish further treatment and/or tests
Termination of project	Data collection terminated at end of funding period

significant factor in recovery. To avoid etiology as a confounding variable, only subjects with a single unilateral cerebrovascular accident (CVA) were included. Therefore, this included infarcts and stable intracerebral hemorrhages. Excluded were those subjects with hemorrhages due to arterio-venous malfunction, aneurysm rupture, or subarachnoid hemorrhages. Any person who completely recovered language skills within 5 days of onset was considered to have had a TIA and was excluded.

The goal of the study was to examine treatment effects. Therefore, subjects with unstable medical illnesses, such as congestive heart failure, which interfered with testing or survival, were excluded. To ensure that all subjects were able to take advantage of treatment, hearing impaired or blind individuals were excluded. Subjects had to demonstrate age-appropriate hearing sensitivity aided or unaided in at least one ear for the speech frequencies 500, 1000, and 2000 Hz. Blindness was defined clinically as a visual impairment sufficiently severe to interfere with seeing the test materials adequately. Blind subjects were also excluded from the investigation because visual limitations would interfere with the normal conduct of treatment. Because integrity of the tactile system was not crucial to either test performance or treatment performance, tactile dysfunction was not a cause of exclusion.

Only subjects who were tested within 2 to 4 weeks post stroke were eligible to participate, and any subject who received an Aphasia Quotient (AQ) of 93.8 or above on initial testing with the Western Aphasia Battery (WAB) (Kertesz and Poole, 1974) was excluded. Since testing and treatment were available only in English, the population included only routine speakers of English for whom treatment was appropriate in English.

A subject who met all the entry criteria was scheduled for initial testing. Results of this initial WAB testing were used to classify the patient for type and severity of aphasia (Table 12–3). Subjects were accepted who fell within the categories of global, Broca's, Wernicke's, anomic, and conduction aphasia as defined taxonomically by the WAB. Table 12–4 represents the pattern of score ranges on fluency, auditory comprehension, repetition, and naming, which are used to define these categories of aphasia. Subjects spanned all severity levels from mild to severe. These severity levels were assigned using each aphasic subject's initial WAB AQ score. Table 12–5 shows the score ranges for mild, moderate, and severe levels, established with the original WAB standardization group, for five types of aphasia.

Subjects in the large recovery study were randomly assigned to a treatment group. Therefore, there were no selection factors operating in the assignment of subjects to LOT. However, in order to preserve a balanced subject group, randomization was stratified for type and severity of aphasia.

As a result of these procedures, 28 subjects were assigned to receive LOT. Examination of initial data revealed that the hemorrhage patients were not similar to the infarct patients; therefore, one hemorrhage patient in LOT group was excluded from further analysis and consideration.

Table 12–3. Type and Severity of Aphasia

Type of Aphasia	Severity		
	Mild	Moderate	Severe
Global	—	—	8
Broca's	1	3	3
Wernicke's	2	1	1
Anomic	3	1	—
Conduction	3	1	—
Total	9	6	12

A — sign means that the severity category was not applicable. For example, global aphasic patients are always severe.

Demographic data for the LOT group are shown in Table 12–6. The age range for the group was 29 to 82 years, with a mean of 62.33 and a median of 63.0 years. The shape of the distribution was negatively skewed, with more of the subjects occurring in the older decades. Educational level varied from 4 to 21 years, with a mean of 9.85 years and a median of 9.0 years of formal education. In the Ontario education system, completion of high school takes 13 years; therefore, a ninth grade education represents first-year high school completion.

A measure of socioeconomic status was obtained using the Blishen Scale (Blishen and McRoberts, 1976). This scale assigns a socioeconomic index to almost 500 Canadian occupations using a combination of income

Table 12–4. Criteria for Classification*

	Fluency	Comprehension	Repetition	Naming
Global	0–4.0	0–3.94	0–4.9	0–6.9
Broca's	0–4.0	3.95–10.0	0–7.9	0–8.9
Wernicke's	5.0–10.0	0–6.94	0–7.9	0–7.9
Anomic	5.0–10.0	6.95–10.0	7.0–10.0	0–9.9
Conduction	5.0–10.0	6.95–10.0	0–6.9	0–9.9

*Modified from Kertesz, A., and McCabe, P. (1977). Recovery patterns and prognosis in aphasia. Brain, 100, 1–18.

Table 12–5. AQ Score Range for Mild, Moderate, and Severe Levels by Type of Aphasia

Type of Aphasia	AQ Score Range		
	Mild	Moderate	Severe
Global (N = 26)			0–15+*
Broca's (N = 24)	50–69+	30–49	†<10–29
Wernicke's (N = 27)	50–69+	30–49	<10–29
Anomic (N = 40)	79–94	< 64–78	
Conduction (N = 15)	56–78+	< 32–55	

*The plus sign (+) means that a higher score than actually obtained in the standardization group is possible within the severity level. Therefore, a global aphasic patient could obtain a score higher than 15, but none did among the 26 global aphasic patients in the standardization group.

†The < sign means that a lower score than actually obtained in the standardization group is possible within the severity level. Therefore, a moderate conduction aphasic patient could obtain a score lower than 32, but none did among the 15 conduction aphasic subjects in the standardization group.

Table 12–6. Demographic Data for 27 LOT Subjects

Age (Years)	
Mean	62.33
Median	63.0
Range	28–82
Education (Years)	
Mean	9.85
Median	9.0
Range	4–21
Socioeconomic Status	
Mean	38.92
Sex	
Male	17
Female	10
Handedness	
Right	25
Left	1
Ambidextrous	1
Language	
English	22
Polyglot	5
Etiology	
Infarction	27

and educational level factors. The scores for the entire list of occupations range from 19.24 to 75.28. The scores for the LOT subjects spanned almost the entire range, from 24.27 to 72.73, with a mean of 38.92. Because homemaker was not listed as an occupation, the mean score of the entire sample was used for this occupation. The mean score for the older aphasic group was identical to that of a sample of 60 older normal persons (aged 40 to 79 years) collected from the same regional area (Shewan and Henderson, 1984). This would suggest that the socioeconomic status of the aphasic sample did not differ from that of the general population.

The LOT group was composed of 17 male and 10 female aphasic patients. The ratio of 1.7 to 1.0 reflects the greater incidence of stroke and aphasia among males and is in line with previous research reports (Abu-Zeid, Choi, and Nelson, 1975; Kurtzke, 1976). Handedness of subjects, assessed by responses to a questionnaire containing seven questions, was predominantly right handed (N = 25), with one subject each in the left-handed and ambidextrous categories. All subjects received their treatment in the English language. For 22 subjects, this was their only language known. Five subjects spoke two or more languages.

METHODS AND PROCEDURES

Subjects referred to the study who met the entry criteria were tested at systematic test intervals, with the initial test (entry) occurring within 2 to 4 weeks post stroke. Additional tests were administered at 3 months, 6 months, and 12 months after the first test. A followup test was also administered 6 months after treatment had terminated. Each subject was tested individually in a quiet room in a hospital setting. The examiners who administered all tests were trained to administer them reliably and were independent of the clinicians providing treatment.

The test battery administered included the WAB (Kertesz and Poole, 1974), the Auditory Comprehension Test for Sentences (ACTS) (Shewan, 1979), and Raven's Coloured Progressive Matrices (RCPM) (Raven, 1956).

All subjects received a neurological examination at the test intervals described. The presence, side, and severity of hemiplegia was evaluated as well as the presence and side of both hemianopsia and hemisensory loss. Side and site of lesion were confirmed in all cases by computerized tomographic (CT) or isotope brain scan. Neurological data at entry are shown in Table 12-7.

Treatment was initiated as soon as possible after initial testing and always within 7 weeks of onset of aphasia. The number of days post onset ranged from 20 to 47, with a mean of 32.8. Patients were assigned to a clini-

Table 12-7.   Neurological Data for 27 LOT Subjects

Lesion		Hemiplegia				Hemianopsia	Hemisensory Loss
	Side	Severity					
		Mild	Moderate	Severe			
Right	1	17	3	3	11	8	11
Left	26	—	—	—	—	—	—

cian with current caseload and geographical location being the primary variables considered, preventing a totally random assignment. However, no attempt was made to match the patient and clinician.

Treatment for the participants was controlled for duration and intensity. All subjects received 1 year of language treatment unless they exited from the study prior to that time. This served as a control for the duration of treatment. The intensity of treatment was controlled by providing each subject with three 1-hour sessions weekly. In some cases, when travel distance to treatment prohibited this regimen and when the patient could accommodate it, two treatment sessions of 1½ hours were provided. The total amount of treatment for the LOT patients constituted 1492 sessions, with a mean of 55.26 and a range of 1 to 118 sessions. All subjects did not receive the same amount of treatment because some subjects exited from the study prior to completion of treatment. Table 12-8 summarizes the frequency distribution of the number of treatment sessions attended. Exit criteria (Table 12-2) included language recovery, death, occurrence of a second stroke, prolonged illness, geographical relocation, voluntary withdrawal from further participation, or termination of the study. If a patient exited from the study, this patient was lost to further followup. Table 12-9 lists the reasons for loss to followup of the six patients within the first 3 months post onset of aphasia.

Table 12-8.   Frequency Distribution of Attended LOT Treatment Sessions

Number of Sessions	Number of Patients	Percent of Patients
0–25	8	29.6
26–50	6	22.2
51–75	3	11.1
76–100	3	11.1
101–125	7	25.9
Total	27	100.0*

*Percent may not add to 100.0 due to rounding.

Table 12–9. Loss to Followup Patients

Reason	Number	Percent
Death	1	16.67
Medical Problem	—	—
Geographical Relocation	2	33.33
Voluntary Withdrawal	3	50.00

Treatment was provided on an individual basis in a clinical setting. All clinicians were trained professional speech-language pathologists. In addition, each clinician had experience in treating aphasic patients and 83.3 percent ($^{10}/_{12}$) had used LOT under one author's (C. M. Shewan) supervision prior to the study's initiation. One of the remaining clinicians (D. L. Bandur) had assisted in developing LOT and consequently was very familiar with the procedures. To ensure that all clinicians followed LOT as intended, each received an LOT training program. Following this, and prior to providing any LOT treatment, all clinicians demonstrated satisfactory ability to execute LOT both to the trainer (C. M. Shewan) and to an external examiner by completing a case study that required planning LOT for a 1-month period. If both evaluators passed the case study, the clinician was eligible to treat patients. To ensure that all clinicians actually provided LOT throughout the study, at 6-month intervals, their treatment was evaluated by a second external examiner who was unfamiliar with any of the clinicians. For all LOT clinicians at all observations (100 percent), this examiner assigned LOT as the treatment type being provided.

Data were collected, computerized, and stored for each treatment session for each patient as long as treatment continued. Which of the five language modalities were used and the amount of time spent in treatment was recorded. In addition, which areas within each modality were used and the percentage correct responses for each area were recorded. It was, therefore, possible to determine the pattern of treatment for a particular session and to obtain a pattern across sessions (time) for patients, individually and collectively.

EFFICACY OF LOT

To demonstrate the efficacy of LOT, this subject group was compared with a control group who had not received treatment.[1] The control group included 22 subjects who met the entry criteria and who did not wish or who

---

[1]The results of the larger study are reported in Shewan and Kertesz (1984).

were unable to receive treatment. The no-treatment control (NTC) group was comparable with the LOT group for age, education, socioeconomic status, handedness, language, and etiology. However, sex distribution was different, as the number of males (N = 11) and females (N = 11) was equal. Ethical considerations did not permit randomization to this group.

Whether LOT had significant positive effects was examined using analysis of covariance, controlling for initial severity of language impairment. The outcome of measures of interest were (1) the Language Quotient (LQ) of the WAB, a composite index of the oral and written language subtests (Spontaneous Speech, Auditory Comprehension, Repetition, Naming, Reading, and Writing) and (2) the Cortical Quotient (CQ) of the WAB, a summary index of cortical functioning that adds Praxis and Construction subtests to those for language. The dependent variable in the analyses was the WAB LQ or CQ on the last test for each subject, referred to as the LQLAST or CQLAST. It was necessary to control for the WAB entry score in the analyses, since it reflected the initial severity level of the patient, a variable known to influence final outcome (Butfield and Zangwill, 1946; Dabul and Hanson, 1975; Keenan and Brassell, 1974; Schuell et al., 1964). Difference scores between the entry test and the last test could not be used in the data analyses because the higher entry scores of the control group created an imbalance between the groups and the degree of change in the outcome measure was related to the entry score (Lee, 1980).

Because some patients were lost to followup prior to receiving the full year of treatment, the data analysis was limited to subjects who had received an entry test battery and at least one additional battery at 3 months, 6 months, or 12 months post onset. These analyses did include all subjects who recovered during this time period.

The LQLAST was used as the dependent variable in an analysis of covariance. Results shown in Table 12–10 indicated that treatment (LOT) had significant positive effects compared with no treatment. The estimate of the difference between the LOT and control group means, after adjusting for entry score and educational level, was 11.50, with a standard error of 4.71 (p<.02). After considering other possible variables which might influence results, age (18 to 59 versus 60 to 85 year groups) and sex were added as concomitant variables to the analysis of covariance. The results were essentially unchanged; therefore, subsequent analyses did not control for these variables.

Similar analyses were carried out using the CQ of the WAB as the outcome measure, as it was reasoned that treatment might have a more generalized effect on recovery and the CQ is purported to measure general cortical functioning. Because the initial testing was carried out during the early period post stroke, all subjects were unable to complete the entire test battery. Therefore, the numbers in the LOT and NTC groups were 16 and

Table 12–10. Summary of Analyses of Covariance for LQ and CQ Outcome Measures for LOT and NTC Groups

	LQ			CQ	
p	Estimate of Adjusted Mean Difference	Standard Error	p	Estimate of Adjusted Mean Difference	Standard Error
≤.02	11.50	Entry — Last Test 4.75	≤.07	8.27	4.35
≤.43	3.93	Entry — Test 2 4.90	≤.49	−2.71	3.85
≤.02	5.86	Test 2 — Last Test 2.19	≤.15	4.04	2.65

14, respectively. With this comparison, the differences between the LOT and NTC groups did not reach significance (p>.07) but approached it. Therefore, LOT treatment appeared to have its greatest effects on language recovery rather than on more generalized recovery of both language and nonlanguage aspects.

When examining the effects of language treatment it is important to control for spontaneous recovery. Therefore, the next step in the data analysis did control for this by determining when treatment had its greatest effects. Including all subjects who received each test, that is, using cross-sectional data, can be misleading because those subjects who remain in a clinical trial may not be representative of all subjects at entry. From the LOT and NTC subjects at entry, 21 remained at least 6 months. Their data were divided into two time intervals: Entry to Test 2 (3 months after the first test), the period most frequently associated with spontaneous recovery, and Test 2 to Last Test (6 or 12 months after the first test). Table 12–10 shows the results of the analyses of covariance. During the early phase corresponding to the spontaneous recovery period, both groups performed similarly and both made gains. This was true for both the LQ and CQ outcome measures. For the late phase, however, LQ gains were significantly greater in the LOT group than in the NTC group (p ≤.02). They were not significant for the CQ measure (p ≤.15). This again suggested that the effects of LOT treatment were more beneficial for language functioning than for more generalized functioning, which included nonlanguage behaviors.

The number of aphasic patients corresponding to each type of aphasia was too small to permit statistical analyses. However, it was profitable to examine the recovery curves for each type to determine how recovery took place and to examine the recovery within each type. Because the number of subjects who contributed to the mean score at each test was potentially different due to patients lost to followup, the patients were grouped according to the number of tests they received, and the mean scores for each group, referred to as streams, are shown (Fig. 12–1).

Looking at the streams in the total LOT group it can be seen that LQ scores increased as time elapsed. For streams that remained in the study for two or more tests, the greatest gains were made in the first 3 months, with fewer but substantial gains until treatment terminated. For the most part, these gains were maintained after treatment terminated, as the Test 5 mean LQ score (6 months after termination of treatment) was only 1.4 points below the Test 4 mean score.

For the global aphasic group, gains were seen for the first 6 months, and then stabilization occurred for the three patients who remained in the study. The LQ gain of 20 points from Entry to Test 4 was comparable with that for the entire LOT group. However, the global group both started and finished with lower scores. After termination of treatment, the gains achieved were maintained for at least a 6-month period.

The Broca's aphasic group showed gains throughout the course of treatment. They made substantial gains during the second 6 months of treatment and declined only slightly when treatment terminated (2.4 points).

With the small number of Wernicke's patients in the group and with only one remaining beyond 3 months, results are speculative. This remaining patient also started out with a less severe impairment than the group as a whole. His pattern was one of a negatively accelerated curve with a peak at the termination of treatment, followed by a slight decline over the 6-month followup period.

In general, the anomic group was less severe than the nonfluent groups at entry. However, they did make LQ gains in the neighborhood of 20 points. Although the greatest gains occurred in the first 3 months, gains were seen for both the 3- to 6-month and 6- to 12-month periods. Unfortunately, no followup tests were available for anomic patients.

Of the four patients in the conduction group, two remained for 6 months of treatment. The greatest gains were seen in the first 3 months and the two remaining patients were approaching complete recovery ($LQ \geq 94.0$) at their 6-month test. No further data were available.

The pattern of recovery was similarly examined for LOT patients divided into mild, moderate, and severe groups on the basis of their initial test battery (Fig. 12–2). The mild group gained an average of 24.8 points on the LQ during treatment. The greatest gains occurred in the first 3 months, although gains were also seen in the next two stages. A slight decline was noticed in the followup phase, although only one patient was available for testing.

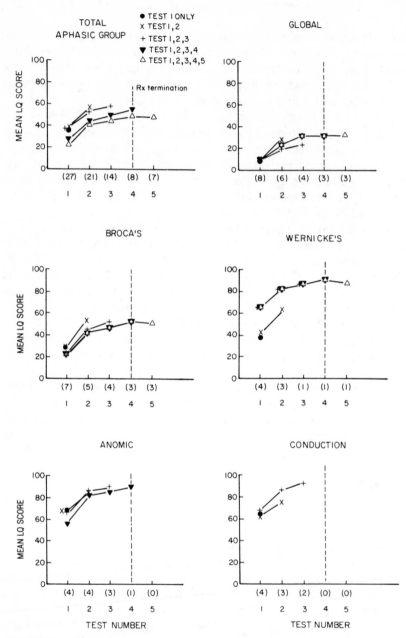

Figure 12–1. Mean LQ scores at Tests 1, 2, 3, 4, and 5 for the total LOT group and the five types of aphasia: global, Broca's, Wernicke's, anomic, and conduction. Patients have been grouped. into streams according to the number of tests received. The numbers in parentheses refer to the number of patients included at each test. Termination of treatment (Rx termination) is represented with a dashed line. Test 5 is a followup test 6 months after treatment terminated.

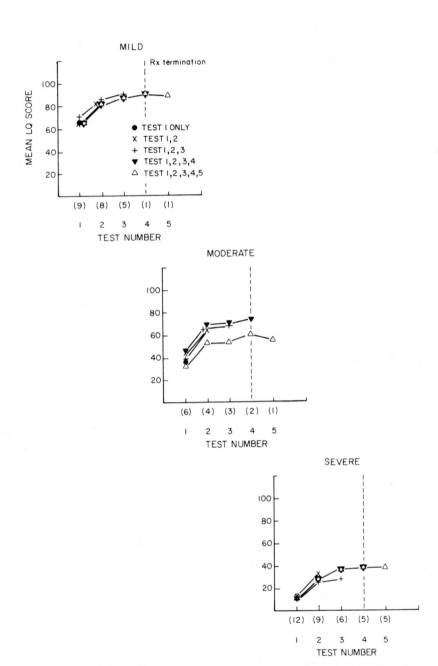

Figure 12–2. Mean LQ scores at Tests 1, 2, 3, 4, and 5 for the mild, moderate, and severe groups. Patients have been grouped into streams according to the number of tests received. The numbers in parentheses refer to the number of patients included at each test. Termination of treatment (Rx termination) is represented with a dashed line. Test 5 is a followup test 6 months after treatment terminated.

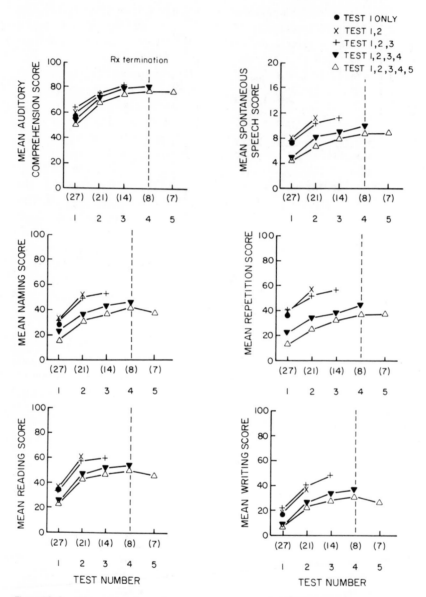

Figure 12–3. Mean scores for auditory comprehension, spontaneous speech, naming, repetition, reading, and writing LQ subtests at Tests 1, 2, 3, 4, and 5 for LOT group. Patients have been grouped into streams according to the number of tests received. The numbers in parentheses refer to the number of patients included at each test. The auditory comprehension scores were divided by two to make them more comparable with other students. Termination of treatment (Rx termination) is represented with a dashed line. Test 5 is a followup test 6 months after treatment terminated.

The moderate group gained an average of 33.8 points on the LQ. The group gained substantially in the first 3 months, only slightly in the next 3 months, and moderately in the last 6 months. The one patient at followup showed a moderate decline from the termination of treatment.

The gain for the severe group of 24.7 points on the LQ was comparable with that for the mild group. As for the other groups, their greatest gains were in the first 3 months. Gains were seen in the second 3-month period, after which only slight gains occurred. The patients who were available for followup testing remained stable after treatment had terminated.

In addition to the LQ summary score, recovery trends were examined for each subtest contained in the LQ (Fig. 12–3). Consistent with that analysis, the patient groups were divided into streams according to the number of tests that had been received. To make the auditory comprehension scores more directly comparable with other subtests, they were divided by two, yielding range scores of 0 to 100.

When the data were examined across time, the greatest amount of recovery occurred in the first 3 months for all subtests and for all streams of patients. Additional gains consistently accrued during each remaining treatment period although they tended to be smaller with increasing time after onset. A followup test 6 months after treatment terminated showed that the treatment gains were maintained for auditory comprehension, spontaneous speech, and repetition. The performance decrements seen for naming, reading, and writing ranged from 2.6 to 3.6 points. They reduced performance to levels close to those seen at Test 3. Since the number of LOT patients who remained throughout the entire time period was small (N = 7), these results are suggestive only. Further data are needed to determine their reliability and generalizability across types and severities of aphasia.

Chapter 13

A Description of LOT Administered to Aphasic Individuals

Chapter 12 provided evidence that the patients who received LOT made language recovery gains in their overall LQ scores and in all individual language subtests. Although this information subtantiates that language treatment and language recovery go hand in hand, the clinician interested in practicing LOT would benefit from more specific and detailed data about the content of treatment. It is the goal of this chapter to describe the major characteristics of LOT treatment, using as a data base the results of its administration to a group of aphasic patients described previously. This description starts by examining which modalities were selected for treatment and which areas within these modalities contributed to treatment. Information about average amount of treatment time spent as well as if and how treatment changed across sessions is included. Describing the treatment profiles separately for each type and severity of aphasia provides prototypes that can be used as the basis for developing each individualized treatment plan.

OVERALL COMPOSITION OF LOT

The content of LOT was divided into five language modalities outlined earlier. The percentage of all treatment sessions that included each language modality is shown in Table 13–1. These percentages provided a

Table 13-1.   Percentage of Treatment Sessions and Percentage of Total Responses by Modality

Modality	Percentage of Treatment Sessions	Percentage of Total Responses
Auditory processing	54.8	21.8
Visual processing	57.1	22.7
Gestural and gestural-verbal communication	13.1	5.2
Oral expression	78.2	31.1
Graphic expression	48.6	19.3
Total		100.0*

*Total may not add to 100.0 due to rounding.

rank ordering from most frequent to least frequent of oral expression, visual processing, auditory processing, graphic expression, and gestural and gestural-verbal communication. As might be expected the spoken language modalities appeared in a large percentage of the sessions, 54.8 percent for auditory processing and 78.2 percent for oral expression. These accounted for 52.9 percent of all treatment occurrences, that is, the occurrence of treatment summed across all five modalities. This high frequency would appear to coincide with the greater relative frequency of spoken language occurrences in everyday life (Chédru and Geschwind, 1972). Visual processing and graphic expression were treated in 57.1 and 48.6 percent of the treatment sessions, that is, approximately half the sessions included these modalities. Gestural training occurred in 13.1 percent of the treatment sessions, representing 5.2 percent of the total treatment occurrences.

A second important dimension of treatment, in addition to its frequency, is the amount of time devoted to each modality. For each session that a patient was treated in and modality the amount of time spent was recorded in minutes. Examination of the relative times across the five modalities showed that the mean time (Table 13-2) closely paralleled that for the frequency of treatment. The one difference was the reversal between auditory processing and graphic expression. The total time for each modality was divided by the number of sessions in which treatment in the modality took place to yield a mean time per session. Table 13-2 shows that the largest mean time occurred for oral expression (23.0 min) followed by graphic expression (17.2 min). Although the frequency of treatment was almost the lowest for the graphic expression modality, when it was trained, the clinicians spent almost one third of the treatment session for these activities. This may be a reflection, in part, that writing is slow for aphasic patients and these activities require a relatively longer period of time to complete than those for other modalities.

Table 13-2. Treatment Time Overall and Mean Time per Session by Language Modality

Modality	Total Time (Minutes)	Percentage of Total Time	Mean Time per Treated Session (Minutes)
Auditory processing	12,417	18.34	15.18
Visual processing	13,218	19.53	15.51
Gestural and gestural-verbal Communication	2,798	4.13	14.28
Oral expression	26,795	39.59	22.96
Graphic expression	12,461	18.41	17.19

Because of the large number of treatment sessions (N = 1492), examining the nature of treatment across time, that is, across treatment sessions, required analyzing the data from more than one session simultaneously. At a frequency of 3 sessions per week, each month encompassed approximately 14 treatment sessions. Therefore, this class interval was selected as the unit to be used in the data analysis. This procedure facilitated the detection of patterns or trends present in the data.

An important question was whether, for treatment in general, the frequency of treatment within modalities changed across time. For example, did the majority of auditory processing training occur early with very little occurring later in treatment? Because the number of subjects receiving treatment changed across time, the data have been reported using mean frequency and mean time values. The mean frequency represents the average number of sessions, from the possible interval of 14 sessions, that a subject received treatment in a particular modality. It is important to recall that the overall frequency of treatment in the five modalities differed. From Table 13-3, accounting for minor fluctuations, the mean treatment frequency for auditory processing was 7, or half the possible sessions, and relatively constant for the first 9 intervals. The frequency dropped to approximately 3 during the last 3 intervals. The mean frequency for visual processing was relatively constant across time, and this modality was included for approximately 7 of the possible 14 sessions in each interval. Treatment for the gestural and gestural-verbal communication modality was concentrated in the middle treatment intervals, and for only 3 of the 12 did the mean frequency reach 7. Frequency of treatment was low in both the initial and in the final treatment months. The mean frequency for oral expression was relatively constant across time and the highest of all five modalities. Treatment occurred for greater than half the 14 sessions in 10 of the 12 time intervals. The occurrence of training in graphic expression was also relatively constant across time, indicating that this modality received attention throughout the course of treatment. The mean fre-

Table 13–3. Mean Frequency and Mean Time of Treatment for Five Modalities Grouped According to Treatment Intervals of Fourteen Sessions

Treatment Sessions	Language Modality									
	Auditory Processing		Visual Processing		Gestural and Gestural-Verbal Communication*		Oral Expression		Graphic Expression	
	Frequency†	Time‡	Frequency	Time	Frequency	Time	Frequency	Time	Frequency	Time
1–14	6.6	100.3	6.9	98.5	3.8	25.0	8.5	194.0	6.0	88.6
15–28	9.5	136.6	7.9	113.0	1.0	7.5	9.9	234.1	7.9	127.9
29–42	5.5	83.2	6.1	109.8	5.5	72.5	6.7	156.6	4.7	84.4
43–56	6.3	95.8	7.1	115.2	5.5	95.5	8.6	200.7	6.6	123.6
57–70	7.3	102.5	6.9	103.5	9.7	111.7	8.5	202.3	8.5	199.1
71–84	6.1	100.1	4.8	71.7	8.0	199.0	6.9	145.4	4.8	81.0
85–98	7.1	118.1	6.3	106.8	4.8	38.3	8.4	183.4	6.7	125.4
99–112	7.0	109.6	7.3	109.7	6.8	88.0	8.2	212.5	6.4	101.7
113–126	7.6	125.0	6.9	107.8	6.0	93.2	8.1	163.6	7.2	102.3
127–140	5.0	71.2	6.4	100.4	8.7	151.0	8.2	167.8	5.2	95.4
141–154	5.0	57.3	6.2	116.3	5.0	95.0	7.3	145.8	5.0	78.2
155–168	0.0	0.0	7.0	62.0	0.0	0.0	7.0	178.0	6.0	105.0

*Only 5 subjects received any training in this modality.
†The mean frequency has a possible range from 0 to 14.
‡The mean time has a possible range from 0 to 840. If each of the 14 sessions treated a single modality for all 60 minutes, the total is 840 minutes per subject.

quencies were similar to those for auditory processing and visual processing modalities. Because graphic expression was the most impaired modality for all streams of aphasic patients (see the mean writing scores in Fig. 12–3), and because it has been reported to recover the latest and the least of the language modalities, it was anticipated that training in this modality might have been less frequent and might have occurred only in the later treatment stages. However, this was not the case.

The mean treatment time (in minutes) for each interval of 14 sessions for each language modality is shown in Table 13–3. Naturally, the mean times values are larger than the mean frequencies; however, they follow the same pattern for all five modalities. These patterns are shown in Figure 13–1.

RELATIVE CONTRIBUTION TO TREATMENT OF EACH AREA TO ITS RESPECTIVE LANGUAGE MODALITY

In addition to knowing which modalities were used in treatment and the general pattern of that treatment, it was also instructive to examine which areas contributed to the treatment within each modality. As previously, each modality was examined separately, and the percentage contribution of each area within each modality is shown in Figure 13–2.

The division of the auditory processing modality into perceptual and comprehension components was reflected in the treatment provided. That few aphasic patients demonstrate auditory perceptual problems was discussed in Chapter 2 and treatment in these three areas accounted for only 6.1 percent of the modality total. Auditory comprehension training, therefore, accounted for 93.9 percent of the training. Comprehension of single words and sentences contributed the largest percentages, 20.8 and 42.6 percent, respectively.

The perceptual category of the visual processing modality comprises three areas: matching nonverbal material, matching verbal material, and visual correspondence. These areas accounted for 30.2 percent of the treatment in this modality. Within the comprehension category, two areas, reading comprehension and reading textual material, were treated most frequently, composing 65.9 percent of the total training. Almost no communication to the patients was via gesture alone (0.66 percent), although gesture may have been used as a supporting cue to auditory presentation.

Treatment in communication via gesture or gesture plus verbalization was used less than treatment in the other modalities. However, within this modality training concentrated on a single area (63.8 percent), entitled gestural communication, the use of single simple gestures for com-

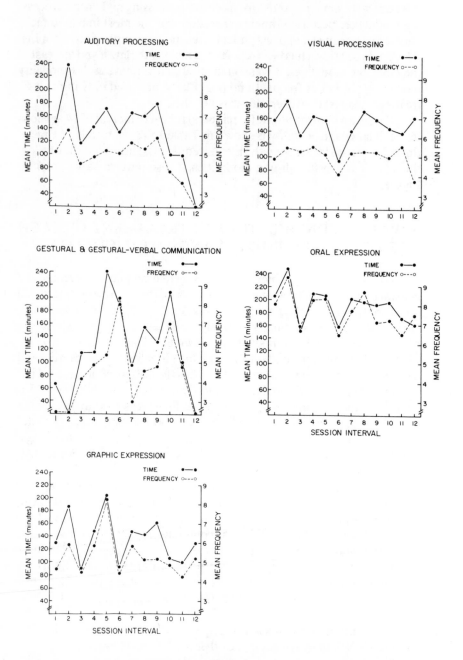

Figure 13–1. Mean treatment time (minutes) and mean frequency of treatment across session intervals for the five treatment modalities.

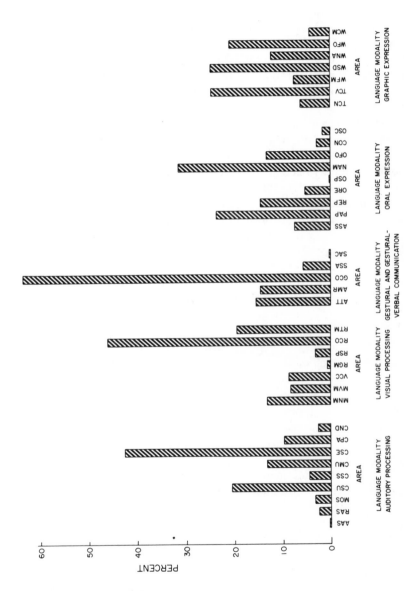

Figure 13–2. Percentage, based on the frequency of treatment, that each area contributed to its respective treatment modality. (See Fig. 1–1 for the complete name of each area).

municating messages. Very little treatment (5.8 percent) extended beyond gesture alone, to areas that included gesture by verbalization. Treatment did encompass gestures used to gain attention and to acknowledge receipt of a message (30.4 percent).

In the oral expression modality, all areas except oral spelling received treatment. As might be expected verbal dyspraxia (23.7 percent), naming (31.3 percent), and repetition (14.7 percent) activities were prominent, accounting for 69.7 percent of the treatment. Within formulation areas, the greatest percentage of treatment (13.2 percent) dealt with oral formulation, the spontaneous production of utterances. Although patients were treated in conversation and extended narratives, these areas occurred as small percentages overall.

Reproduction of verbal and nonverbal material as well as spontaneous production of highly overlearned material contributed 38.6 percent of all graphic expression treatment. Tracing or copying verbal material, or both, at 24.7 percent, was the most frequent activity. Writing dictated words and written naming, training at the single word level, accounted for 24.1 percent and 12.2 percent of treatment. More complex activities involving written formulation completed the remaining 25.1 percent of treatment in this modality, with written formulation being the heavier contributor (20.9 percent).

TREATMENT PROFILES FOR EACH TYPE OF APHASIA

Global Aphasia

For the global aphasic patients, treatment concentrated on three modalities, each of which was included in greater than 65 percent of the sessions (Table 13–4). Since global aphasic patients are described as being impaired in all language modalities, a pattern of treatment that concentrated on visual processing, oral expression, and auditory comprehension was consistent with their pattern of language deficits. Graphic expression received training in 47.1 percent of the sessions, with 26.9 percent receiving gestural training.

The amount of treatment revealed a similar pattern to the frequency with which treatment took place in each modality (Table 13–5). Thirty percent of the time involved oral expression, followed by 25.1 percent for visual processing and 21.0 percent for auditory processing. Graphic expression (14.1 percent) and gestural and gestural-verbal training (9.1 percent) accounted for less than 25 percent of treatment time overall.

Because this pattern of frequency of treatment across the 12 intervals of sessions generally mirrored treatment time, the data presented will discuss the time dimension only. The time interval data were further consolidated into four periods, each accounting for approximately 3 months

Table 13-4. Percentage of Treatment Sessions Including Each Modality for Five Aphasic Types

Modality	Global (percent)	Broca's (percent)	Wernicke's (percent)	Anomic (percent)	Conduction (percent)
Auditory processing	66.9	65.0	61.7	11.0	41.6
Visual processing	70.9	46.5	60.0	57.8	38.5
Gestural and gestural-verbal communication	26.9	14.1	0.0	0.0	0.0
Oral expression	69.3	89.4	91.7	67.0	76.4
Graphic expression	47.1	30.3	76.7	62.4	52.2

of treatment. For the globals the last period contained only 2 months. The mean amount of auditory processing time decreased over the four periods (Fig. 13–3), whereas visual processing time increased. Gestural and gestural-verbal communication and graphic expression showed initial increases, with later declines. Oral expression started at a higher level than the other modalities, initially increased and later dropped slightly.

Broca's Aphasia

The mean amount of time devoted to auditory processing peaked at Period 3 and declined dramatically for the last period (Fig. 13–3). Visual processing received less time than its auditory counterpart and treatment peaked at Period 2, with successive declines for the remaining two periods. Gestural and gestural-verbal treatment did not appear until Period 2, with very little training even then. There were substantial increases for the remaining two periods, although it never reached the levels for the other expressive modalities. The pattern for oral expression, with treatment at a high level throughout the four periods, was con-

Table 13-5. Treatment Time Overall and Percentage Time for Five Modalities by Type of Aphasia

Modality	Global (N = 8) Total Time (Min)	(%)	Broca's (N = 7) Total Time (Min)	(%)	Wernicke's (N = 4) Total Time (Min)	(%)	Anomic (N = 4) Total Time (Min)	(%)	Conduction (N = 4) Total Time (Min)	(%)
Auditory processing	4653	21.0	5042	25.3	1430	15.5	245	2.5	1047	15.8
Visual processing	5578	25.1	2392	12.0	1499	16.2	2730	28.0	1019	15.4
Gestural and gestural-verbal communication	2008	9.1	790	4.0	0	0.0	0	0.0	0	0.0
Oral expression	6820	30.7	9683	48.6	3628	39.2	3703	38.0	2961	44.8
Graphic Expression	3120	14.1	1986	10.0	2698	29.2	3068	31.5	1589	24.0
Total	22,179		19,893		9,255		9,746		6,616	

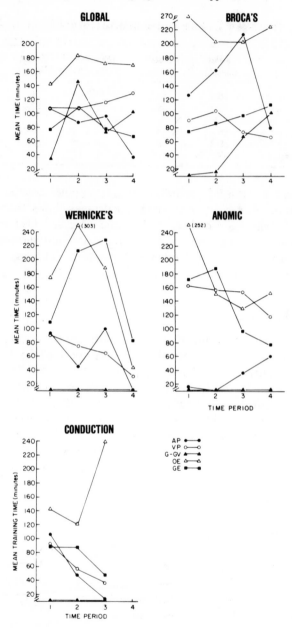

Figure 13-3. Mean treatment time (minutes) based on 14-session intervals for each modality for global, Broca's, Wernicke's, anomic, and conduction aphasia types. Each of the 4 time periods corresponds approximately to 3 months of treatment. AP = Auditory Processing, VP = Visual Processing, G-GV = Gestural and Gestural-Verbal Communication, OE = Oral Expression, GE = Graphic Expression.

vex in shape, with less treatment in the middle two periods. Graphic expression showed a steady rise in treatment time across the four periods. Therefore, the data revealed that the receptive modalities received less treatment over time, whereas the expressive modalities received more.

Wernicke's Aphasia

Because the Wernicke's aphasic group was small, starting with four subjects, which reduced to a single subject for the last two periods, the data presented are considered suggestive only. Somewhat surprising was the small amount of auditory processing treatment; of the treated modalities, it received the smallest amount overall. Perhaps influential was that two of the four patients were of mild severity, with one each in the moderate and severe categories. The majority of the treatment was devoted to the expressive modalities, oral (39.2 percent) and graphic (29.2 percent). No gestural treatment occurred with this group.

The pattern of treatment across time was variable. Auditory processing dropped to half its initial level at Period 2, climbed to slightly beyond its intitial level, and fell to 0 at Period 4. Visual processing started at a level similar to auditory processing and gradually declined across time. Oral expression treatment was initiated at the highest level, rose dramatically in Period 2, and subsequently declined for both successive periods. Graphic expression also showed dramatic shifts across time, rising to a peak during Period 3 and falling substantially thereafter.

Anomic Aphasia

The anomic aphasic group initially comprised four subjects. None of these received more than 10 months' treatment and beyond 6 months, only one subject remained. Therefore, the same cautions apply to the data interpretation as for the Wernicke's group. The rank ordering for frequency and amount of treatment time paralleled one another. Treatment in oral (38.0 percent) and graphic (31.5 percent) expression consumed the most time, followed closely by visual processing (28.0 percent). Little treatment occurred for auditory processing (2.5 percent), consistent with the pattern of language impairment for this group. Consistent with all the fluent aphasic types, no treatment took place in gestural and gestural-verbal communication.

When auditory processing treatment occurred, it generally occurred later and was limited to one subject. Visual processing received more treatment than its auditory counterpart. The amount was relatively constant until the last period, when a noticeable decrement was seen. Oral expression started at a very high level, decreased markedly for the next two periods, and then increased noticeably again. Graphic expression treatment peaked at Period 2, dropped substantially at Period 3, and declined slightly again at Period 4.

Conduction Aphasia

The conduction aphasia group also comprised four subjects. Because they remained in the study for only 9 months, no data were available for Period 4. The small group size warrants a reminder for cautious data interpretation, as with the other fluent groups. Consistent with the anomic group, frequency and amount of treatment time paralleled one another. Oral expression ranked highest for treatment (44.8 percent). Second in rank but with considerably less treatment was graphic expression (24.0 percent). Auditory processing and visual processing received similar amounts of treatment at 15.8 and 15.4 percent, respectively. This group was not treated in gestural and gestural-verbal communication.

The mean time for auditory processing decreased to almost 0 across the three periods (Fig. 13–3). Visual processing showed a similar pattern although its endpoint was not as low as that for auditory processing. Oral expression was consistently treated the most; after a slight decrement from Period 1 to 2, treatment rose sharply during the remaining time. Graphic expression treatment was constant for Periods 1 and 2, followed with a decrement for Period 3.

To compare treatment across aphasia types, each treatment modality was rank ordered from most to least training time for each type of aphasia. Kendall's coefficient of concordance, computed across the five groups, was .808, significant at the .01 level. This indicated that there was a significant relationship in the amount of treatment for the modalities across types of aphasia. For example, for all five types the least treatment was in gestural and gestural-verbal communication and the most treatment was in oral expression. In general, treatment time seemed to parallel the nature of the linguistic deficit for each type of aphasia. The global aphasic group, impaired in all modalities, received large amounts of time for spoken and written language as well as some treatment for gestural communication. Broca's aphasic patients' treatment concentrated on their oral expressive problems. Severe patients in this group also received some gestural treatment. Its later appearance suggested that it occurred as a result of insufficient gains in oral expression. Auditory processing activities comprised 25 percent of the treatment, perhaps more than expected because Broca's aphasic persons have been frequently described as having intact auditory comprehension. Oral expression was heavily emphasized in the Wernicke's group; however, relatively little time (15.5 percent) was devoted to auditory comprehension tasks, perhaps related to the presence of two mild subjects who required little work in this area. As was true for all the fluent types, this group had sufficient verbal output so as not to require gestural treatment. Anomic aphasic patients, as expected, received little work with auditory comprehension. Treatment focused on oral expression and graphic expression, with reading comprehension work as well. The conduction group showed a treatment pattern similar to the Wernicke's group. They received most treatment in oral expression and only a moderate amount in auditory processing.

For all groups of patients the written language modalities accounted for an average of 20.6 percent of the treatment, which occurred throughout the intervals and was not restricted only to the last intervals. Previously reported significant gains in reading and writing (Hagen, 1973) may well be related to the quantity and consistency of treatment in these modalities. The amount of auditory comprehension treatment in comparison with other modalities was smaller than expected, ranking fourth overall. This may reflect the relatively higher initial performance in this modality and its earlier recovery (see Fig. 12–3).

THE NATURE OF TREATMENT FOR DIFFERENT SEVERITY GROUPS

Because different severity groups recover to different degrees and because their problems are different, at least quantitatively, it was important to examine the nature of treatment in different severity groups.

Mild Aphasia

In the mild aphasia group, the greatest percentage of sessions involved the expressive modalities (Table 13–6). Oral expression was included in 77.7 percent and graphic expression in 62.0 percent of treatment sessions. Treatment in visual processing took place in a greater percentage (45.5) of sessions than auditory processing (36.1). No treatment occurred for the gestural and gestural-verbal communication modality.

The rank order for the amount of treatment (time in minutes) paralleled the rank order for frequency just described (Table 13–7). Most time was spent with oral and graphic expression, less for visual and auditory processing, and none for gestural communication.

The pattern of treatment for the four trained modalities was examined across sessions, using the four time periods as described earlier (Fig. 13–4). Auditory and visual processing showed similar patterns, with a decrement at Period 2 and an increase at Period 3 followed by a substantial decline. Oral and graphic expression increased to a peak at Period 3 and decreased

Table 13-6. Percentage of Treatment Sessions Including Each Modality for Three Severity Groups

Modality	Mild (percent)	Moderate (percent)	Severe (percent)
Auditory processing	36.1	65.6	61.5
Visual processing	45.5	72.4	57.9
Gestural and gestural-verbal communication	0.0	0.0	25.9
Oral expression	77.7	86.7	75.2
Graphic expression	62.0	33.3	46.7

in a marked decline at Period 4. To some extent the declines at Period 4 may have reflected the variability in the absolute number of treatment sessions in the last interval of 14 sessions. If a subject received any training in this interval, these data were included. Therefore, there were fewer actual sessions here than for previous intervals.

Moderate Aphasia

The moderate aphasia group contained six subjects initially, which was reduced to two by the end of the treatment period. Oral expression, visual processing, and auditory processing were all included in 65 percent or more of the sessions, with treatment in graphic expression in one third of the sessions. No treatment in gestural or gestural-verbal communication took place, presumably because these patients could rely on verbal means to communicate their messages.

The rank order for percentage of time devoted to each modality paralleled that for frequency. Most time overall was spent with oral expres-

Table 13-7. Treatment Time Overall and Percentage Time for Five Modalities by Severity of Aphasia

Modality	Severity of Aphasia					
	Mild (N = 9) Total Time		Moderate (N = 6) Total Time		Severe (N = 12) Total Time	
	(Min)	(%)	(Min)	(%)	(Min)	(%)
Auditory processing	2115	10.5	3226	24.1	7076	20.7
Visual processing	3214	15.9	3452	25.8	6552	19.2
Gestural and gestural-verbal communication	0	0	0	0	2798	8.2
Oral expression	8704	43.2	5335	39.8	12,756	37.4
Graphic Expression	6127	30.4	1375	10.3	4959	14.5
Total	20,160		13,388		34,141	

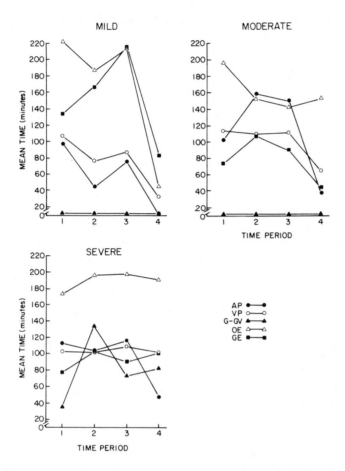

Figure 13–4. Mean treatment time (minutes) based on 14-session intervals for each modality for mild, moderate, and severe aphasia groups. Each of the four time periods corresponds approximately to 3 months of treatment. AP = Auditory Processing, VP = Visual Processing, G-GV = Gestural and Gestural-Verbal Communication, OE = Oral Expression, GE = Graphic Expression.

sion areas and less, but approximately equal amounts, for visual and auditory processing (see Table 13–7).

Across treatment sessions, auditory processing increased to a peak at Period 2, declined slightly at Period 3, and declined markedly at Period 4. Visual processing varied little from its initial position until Period 4, where a noticeable decline was present. The patterns for the expressive modalities were different from one another. Oral expression started at the highest level of all modalities, dropped during Periods 2 and 3, and increased slightly at Period 4. By contrast, graphic expression increased from its initially low level to a peak at Period 2 and was followed by increasingly greater declines at Periods 3 and 4.

Severe Aphasia

The severe aphasia group contained 12 subjects initially, and of course, all the global aphasic patients. These subjects tended to remain longer in treatment, the full 12 intervals.

Treatment occurred in all five modalities, with oral expression and auditory processing being represented most often (Table 13–6). The written language modalities (reading and writing) ranked next in frequency, followed by the gestural and gestural-verbal communication modality. The amount of treatment time paralleled the frequency data (Table 13–7).

Auditory processing time remained relatively constant across the first 3 periods, and decreased noticeably at the fourth. Visual processing remained constant for all periods. Oral expression received the greatest time allotment and, after an initial decrease to Period 2, plateaued at a consistent level. Graphic expression varied slightly across the time periods, initially increasing, declining, and then increasing once again. The increase-decline pattern was similar for gestural and gestural-verbal communication although the shifts tended to be greater.

Evident from the descriptions for each severity group is that their treatment patterns were not identical, although some similarities existed. The rank order of the mean treatment time for the five modalities was similar for mild, moderate, and severe groups. Kendall's coefficient of concordance (W = .822) was significant (p = .04).

The mild and moderate groups received no gestural and gestural-verbal communication treatment, whereas this accounted for 8.2 percent for the severe group. This would seem to indicate that because the less severe groups can rely on verbal skills they do not require an alternate communication method. Treatment for oral expression took place the most in all three groups, accounting for approximately 40 percent of all training. However, the distribution of this treatment was different for the groups. Treatment in graphic expression occurred most in the mild group, which may have been related to their higher initial WAB score in this modality (40) and their consequent ability to perform writing tasks. The moderate and severe groups, with their low initial WAB writing scores (10, 2) may have been less capable of writing performance. Another possible explanation may be the strong motivation of patients to talk as their primary expressive modality. For those who have especial difficulty in this modality, early treatment may have emphasized oral expression. However, Figure 13–4 does not substantiate this explanation because oral expres-

Table 13-8. Mean LQ Difference Scores for Low and High Treatment Groups

Severity	Treatment	
	Low	High
Mild-Moderate	16.07	31.34
Severe	29.10	20.78

sion treatment was high for all three severity levels. The tradeoff appeared to be with the receptive modalities, which initially took more treatment time, thereby leaving less for graphic expression. Within each severity group, auditory and visual processing received approximately the same amounts of treatment, varying only 1.7 percent for the moderate and severe groups and 5.4 percent for the mild group. The moderate group received the most treatment, on the average, compared with the severe and mild groups.

RELATIONSHIP BETWEEN TREATMENT AND LANGUAGE RECOVERY

In Chapter 7, we indicated that LOT treatment was efficacious. To examine the nature of the relationship between treatment and the amount of language recovery, the LOT group was divided into mild, moderate, and severe groups. Within each severity group, subjects were divided according to whether they received a low or high amount of treatment. Those with a low amount of treatment had received less than the LOT group mean and those with a high amount received more than the group mean. The group mean was 2508 minutes, equivalent to fifty 50-minute treatment sessions. The amount of language recovery was measured by the LQ difference between a subject's last LQ test and entry LQ test. Because this division resulted in only one subject in the low moderate category, the mild and moderates were collapsed into one group. Table 13-8 shows the mean LQ gain scores for the resultant four groups. Comparisons between low and high treatment for each severity group revealed a significant difference for the mild-moderate group ($p < .05$). The mean LQ gain was greater for low treatment in the severe group although the difference was not statistically significant. This unexpected result was explained by one subject in the low severe group who gained the greatest amount of all subjects (50.6 points), 13.2 points more than the next closest patient. Eliminating the outlier resulted in a mean score of 18.4 for the low severe group.

References

Abu-Zeid, H. A. H., Choi, N. W., and Nelson, N. A. (1975). Epidemiologic features of cerebrovascular disease in Manitoba: Incidence by age, sex and residence, with etiologic implications. *Canadian Medical Association Journal, 113,* 379–384.

Ajax, E. T. (1967). Dyslexia without agraphia. *Archives of Neurology, 17,* 645–652.

Ajax, E. T., Schenkenberg, T., and Kosteljanetz, M. (1977). Alexia without agraphia and the inferior splenium. *Neurology, 27,* 685–688.

Albert, M. L., and Bear, D. (1974). Time to understand: A case study of word deafness with reference to the role of time in auditory comprehension. *Brain, 97,* 373–384.

Albert, M. L., Goodglass, H., Helm, N. A., Rubens, A. B., and Alexander, M. P. (1981). Clinical aspects of dysphasia. In G. E. Arnold, F. Winckel, and B. D. Wyke (Eds.), *Disorders of Human Communication 2.* New York: Springer-Verlag.

Albert, M. L., Sparks, R. W., and Helm, N. A. (1973). Melodic intonation therapy for aphasia. *Archives of Neurology, 29,* 130–131.

Albert, M. L., Sparks, R., Von Stockert, T., and Sax, D. (1972). A case of auditory agnosia: Linguistic and non-linguistic processing. *Cortex, 8,* 427–443.

Ansell, B. J., and Flowers, C. R. (November, 1980). *Aphasic adults' use of structural linguistic cues for analysing sentences.* Paper presented at the annual convention of the American Speech-Language-Hearing Association, Detroit.

Aronson, M., Shatin, L., and Cook, J. (1956). Sociopsychotherapeutic approach to the treatment of aphasia. *Journal of Speech and Hearing Disorders, 21,* 325–364.

Backus, O. (1952). The use of a group structure in speech therapy. *Journal of Speech and Hearing Disorders, 17,* 11–122.

Barton, M. I. (1971). Recall of generic properties of words in aphasic patients. *Cortex, 7,* 73–82.

Barton, M., Maruszewski, M., and Urrea, D. (1969). Variations in stimulus context and its effect on word-finding ability in aphasics. *Cortex, 5,* 351–365.

Bass, M. J., Donner, A., and McWhinney, I. R. (1982). The effectiveness of the family physician in hypertension screening and management. *Canadian Family Physician, 28,* 255–258.

Basso, A., Capitani, E., and Vignolo, L. A. (1979). Influence of rehabilitation on language skills in aphasia patients: A controlled study. *Archives of Neurology, 36,* 190–196.

Basso, A., Faglioni, P., and Vignolo, L. A. (1975). Étudée controlée de la rééducation du language dans l'aphasie: Comparaison entre aphasiques traités et non-traités. *Revue Neurologique, 131,* 607–614.

Basso, A., Taborrelli, A., and Vignolo, L. A. (1978). Dissociated disorders of speaking and writing in aphasia. *Journal of Neurology, Neurosurgery, and Psychiatry, 41,* 556–563.

Battig, W. F., and Montague, W. E. (1969). Category norms for verbal items in 56 categories. *Journal of Experimental Psychology, 80,* 1–46.

Beauvois, M. F., and Dérouesné, J. (1981). Lexical or orthographic agraphia. *Brain, 104,* 21–49.

Benson, D. F. (1967). Fluency in aphasia: Correlation with radioactive scan localization. *Cortex, 4,* 373–394.

Benson, D. F. (1977). The third alexia. *Archives of Neurology, 34,* 327–331.

Benson, D. F. (1979a). *Aphasia, alexia, and agraphia.* New York: Churchill Livingstone.

Benson, D. F. (1979b). Neurologic coordinates of anomia. In H. Whitaker and H. A. Whitaker (Eds.), *Studies in neurolinguistics* (Vol. 4, pp. 293–328). New York: Academic Press.

Benson, D. F., Brown, J., and Tomlinson, E. B. (1971). Varieties of alexia. *Neurology, 21,* 951–957.

Benson, D. F., and Geschwind, N. (1969). The alexias. In P. J. Vinken and G. Bruyn (Eds.), *Handbook of clinical neurology* (Vol. 4). Amsterdam: North Holland Publishing Co.

Benson, D. F., and Greenberg, J. P. (1969). Visual form agnosia. *Archives of Neurology, 20,* 82–89.

Benton, A. L., Smith, K. C., and Lang, M. (1972). Stimulus characteristics and object naming in aphasic patients. *Journal of Communication Disorders, 5,* 19–24.

Berman, M., and Peale, L. M. (1967). Self-generated cues: A method for aiding aphasic and apractic patients. *Journal of Speech and Hearing Disorders, 32,* 372–376.

Beukelman, D. R., Yorkston, K. M., and Waugh, P. F. (1980). Communication in severe aphasia: Effectiveness of three instruction modalities. *Archives of Physical Medicine and Rehabilitation, 61,* 248–252.

Bisiach, E. (1966). Perceptual factors in the pathogenesis of anomia. *Cortex, 2,* 90–95.

Blackman, N. (1950). Group psychotherapy with aphasics. *Journal of Nervous and Mental Disorders, 111,* 154–163.

Blackman, N., and Tureen, L. L. (1948). Aphasia—A psychosomatic approach in rehabilitation. *Transactions of the American Neurology Association, 73,* 193–196.

Blishen, B. R., and McRoberts, H. A. (1976). A revised socioeconomic index for occupations in Canada. *Canadian Review of Sociology and Anthropology, 13*, 71–73.

Blockolsky, V. D., Frazer, J. M., Kurn, B. A., and Metz, F. E. (1977). *Peel and put pictures.* Communication Skill Builders (Division of Moyer, Vico, Weston, Ont.).

Blumstein, S. E., Cooper, W. E., Goodglass, H., Statlender, S., and Gottlieb, J. (1980). Production deficits in aphasia: A voice-onset time analysis. *Brain and Language, 9,* 153–170.

Blumstein, S. E., Cooper, W. E., Zurif, E. B., and Caramazza, A. (1977). The perception and production of voice-onset time in aphasia. *Neuropsychologia, 15,* 371–383.

Blumstein, S. E., and Goodglass, H. (1972). The perception of stress as a semantic cue in aphasia. *Journal of Speech and Hearing Research, 15,* 800–806.

Boller, F., and Green, E. (1972). Comprehension in severe aphasia. *Cortex, 8,* 382–394.

Bollinger, R. L., and Stout, C. E. (1976). Response-contingent small-step treatment: Performance-based communication intervention. *Journal of Speech and Hearing Disorders, 41,* 40–51.

Bond, S., Ulatowska, H., Macaluso-Haynes, S., and May, E. (1983). Discourse production in aphasia: Relationship to severity of impairment. In R. H. Brookshire (Ed.), *Clinical aphasiology conference proceedings.* Minneapolis: BRK Publishers.

Bonvillian, J. D., and Friedman, R. J. (1978). Language development in another mode: The acquisition of signs by a brain-damaged adult. *Sign Language Studies, 19,* 111–120.

Boone, D. R., and Friedman, H. R. (1976). Writing in aphasia rehabilitation: cursive vs. manuscript. *Journal of Speech and Hearing Disorders, 41,* 523–529.

Bricker, A. L., Schuell, H. M., and Jenkins, J. J. (1964). Frequency and word length on aphasic spelling errors. *Journal of Speech and Hearing Research, 7,* 183–192.

Broida, H. (1977). Language therapy effects in long term aphasia. *Archives of Physical Medicine and Rehabilitation, 58,* 248–253.

Brookshire, R. H. (1971). Effects of trial time and inter-trial interval on naming by aphasic subjects. *Journal of Communication Disorders, 3,* 289–301.

Brookshire, R. H. (1972). Effects of task difficulty on naming performance of aphasic subjects. *Journal of Speech and Hearing Research, 15,* 551–558.

Brookshire, R. H. (1978). Auditory comprehension and aphasia. In D. F. Johns (Ed.), *Clinical management of neurogenic communicative disorders* (pp. 103–128). Boston: Little, Brown and Company.

Brookshire, R. H., and Nicholas, L. E. (1980). Verification of active and passive sentences by aphasic and nonaphasic subjects. *Journal of Speech and Hearing Research, 23,* 878–893.

Brown, J. W., Leader, B. J., and Blum, C. S. (1983). Hemiplegic writing in severe aphasia. *Brain and Language, 19,* 204–215.

Bub, D., Cancelliere, A., and Kertesz, A. (October, 1982). *The orthographic reading route: Evidence for algorithmic grapheme-phoneme conversion in a surface dyslexia.* Paper presented at the 20th annual meeting of the Academy of Aphasia, Lake Mohonk, NY.

Bub, D., and Kertesz, A. (1982a). Deep agraphia. *Brain and Language, 17,* 146–165.

Bub, D., and Kertesz, A. (1982b). Evidence for lexicographic processing in a patient with preserved written over oral single word naming. *Brain, 105,* 697–717.

Buck, R., and Duffy, R. J. (1980). Nonverbal communication of affect in brain-damaged patients. *Cortex, 16,* 351–362.

Burns, M. S., and Canter, G. J. (1977). Phonemic behavior of aphasic patients with posterior cerebral lesions. *Brain and Language, 4,* 492–507.

Butfield, E., and Zangwill, O. L. (1946). Re-education in aphasia: A review of 70 cases. *Journal of Neurology, Neurosurgery, and Psychiatry, 9,* 75–79.

The Canadian Co-operative Study Group. (1978). A randomized trial of aspirin and sulfurpyrazone in threatened stroke. *The New England Journal of Medicine, 299,* 53–59.

Canter, G. J. (November, 1969). *The influence of primary and secondary verbal apraxia on output disturbances in aphasic syndromes.* Paper presented at the annual convention of the American Speech and Hearing Association, Chicago.

Caramazza, A., Berndt, R. S., Basili, A. G., and Koller, J. J. (1981a). Syntactic processing deficits in aphasia. *Cortex, 17,* 333–347.

Caramazza, A., Berndt, R. S., and Hart, J. (1981b). Agrammatic reading. In F. J. Pirozzolo and M. C. Wittrock (Eds.), *Neuropsychological and cognitive processes in reading.* New York: Academic Press.

Caramazza, A., and Zurif, E. B. (1978). Comprehension of complex sentences in children and aphasics: A test of the regression hypothesis. In A. Caramazza and E. B. Zurif (Eds.), *Language Acquisition and Language Breakdown* (pp. 145–161). Baltimore: Johns Hopkins Press.

Caramazza, A., Zurif, E. B., and Gardner, H. (1978). Sentence memory in aphasia. *Neuropsychologia, 16,* 661–669.

Carpenter, R. L., and Rutherford, D. R. (1973). Acoustic cue discrimination in adult aphasia. *Journal of Speech and Hearing Research, 16,* 534–544.

Carroll, J. B., Davies, P., and Richman, B. (1971). *The American Heritage word frequency book.* Boston: Houghton Mifflin Co.

Chall, D. E., and Chall, J. (1948a). A formula for predicting readability. *Educational Research Bulletin, 27,* 11–20.

Chall, D. E., and Chall, J. (1948b). A formula for predicting readability: Instructions. *Educational Research Bulletin, 27,* 37–54.

Chédru, F., and Geschwind, N. (1972). Writing disturbances in acute confusional states. *Neuropsychologia, 10,* 343–353.

Chen, L. C. (1968). "Talking Hand" for aphasic stroke patients. *Geriatrics, 23,* 145–148.

Chen, L. C. (1971). Manual communication by combined alphabet and gestures. *Archives of Physical Medicine and Rehabilitation, 52,* 381–384.

Cicone, M., Wapner, W., Foldi, N., Zurif, E., and Gardner, H. (1979). The relation between gesture and language in aphasic communication. *Brain and Language, 8,* 324–349.

Cohen, D. N., Salanga, V. D., Hully, W., Steinberg, M. C., and Hardy, R. W. (1976). Alexia without agraphia. *Neurology, 26,* 455–459.

Coltheart, M. (October, 1982). *The alexias.* Paper presented at the 20th annual meeting of the Academy of Aphasia, Lake Mohonk, NY.

Coltheart, M., Patterson, K., and Marshall, J. C. (Eds.). (1980). *Deep dyslexia.* London: Routledge and Kegan Paul.

Corbin, M. L. (1951). Group speech therapy for motor aphasia and dysarthria. *Journal of Speech and Hearing Disorders, 16,* 21–34.

Corlew, M. (October, 1975). *Word variables related to naming and types of aphasia.* Paper presented at the annual convention of the American Speech and Hearing Association, Washington, D.C.

Corlew, M. M., and Nation, J. E. (1975). Characteristics of visual stimuli and naming performance in aphasic adults. *Cortex, 11*, 186–191.

Critchley, M. (1939). *The language of gesture.* London: Arnold.

Cumming, W. J. K., Hurwitz, L. J., and Perl, N. T. (1970). A study of a patient who had alexia without agraphia. *Journal of Neurology, Neurosurgery, and Psychiatry, 33*, 34–39.

Dabul, B., and Hanson, W. R. (October, 1975). *The amount of language improvement in adult aphasics related to early and late treatment.* Paper presented at the annual convention of the American Speech and Hearing Association, Washington, DC.

Damasio, A. R. (1977). Varieties and significance of the alexias. *Archives of Neurology, 34*, 325–326.

Daniloff, J. K., Noll, J. D., Fristoe, M., and Lloyd, L. L. (1982). Gestural recognition in patients with aphasia. *Journal of Speech and Hearing Disorders, 47*, 43–49.

Darley, F. L. (November, 1970). *Apraxia of speech: Definition, description, and appraisal.* Paper presented at the annual convention of the American Speech and Hearing Association, New York.

Darley, F. L. (1972). The efficacy of language rehabilitation in aphasia. *Journal of Speech and Hearing Disorders, 37*, 3–21.

Darley, F. L. (1982). *Aphasia.* Philadelphia: W. B. Saunders Company.

Darley, F. L., Aronson, A. E., and Brown, J. R. (1975). *Motor speech disorders.* Philadelphia: W. B. Saunders Company.

Davis, G. A., and Wilcox, M. J. (1981). Incorporating parameters of natural conversation in aphasia treatment. In R. Chapey (Ed.), *Language intervention strategies in adult aphasia.* Baltimore, MD: Williams & Wilkins.

Davis, L., Foldi, N., Gardner, H., and Zurif, E. (1978). Repetition in the transcortical aphasias. *Brain and Language, 6*, 226–238.

Deal, J. L., and Deal, L. A. (1978). Efficacy of aphasia rehabilitation: Preliminary results. In R. H. Brookshire (Ed.), *Clinical aphasiology conference proceedings* (pp. 66–77). Minneapolis: BRK Publishers.

Deloche, G., Jean-Louis, J., Seron, X. (1979). Study of the temporal variables in the spontaneous speech of five aphasic patients in two situations, interview and description. *Brain and Language, 8*, 241–250.

Deloche, G., and Seron, X. (1981). Sentence understanding and knowledge of the world: Evidences from a sentence-picture matching task performed by aphasic patients. *Brain and Language, 14*, 57–69.

De Renzi, E., Motti, F., and Nichelli, P. (1980). Imitating gestures: A quantitative approach to ideomotor apraxia. *Archives of Neurology, 37*, 6–10.

de Villiers, J. G. (1974). Quantitative aspects of agrammatism in aphasia. *Cortex, 10*, 36–54.

Drummond, S. S., Gallagher, T. M., and Mills, R. H. (1981). Word-retrieval in aphasia: An investigation of semantic complexity. *Cortex, 17*, 63–82.

Drummond, S. S., and Rentschler, G. J. (1981). The efficacy of gestural cueing in dyspraxic word-retrieval responses. *Journal of Communication Disorders, 14*, 287–298.

Duffy, R. J., and Buck, R. W. (1979). A study of the relationship between propositional (pantomime) and subpropositional (facial expression) extraverbal behaviors in aphasics. *Folia Phoniatrica, 31*, 129–136.

Duffy, R. J., and Duffy, J. R. (1981). Three studies of deficits in pantomimic expression and pantomimic recognition in aphasia. *Journal of Speech and Hearing Research, 24*, 70–84.

Duffy, R. J., Duffy, J. R., and Mercaitis, P. A. (1984). Comparison of the performances of a fluent and nonfluent aphasic on a pantomimic referential task. *Brain and Language, 21,* 260–273.

Duffy, R. J., Duffy, J. R., and Pearson, K. (1975). Pantomime recognition in aphasic patients. *Journal of Speech and Hearing Research, 18,* 115–132.

Duffy, R. J., and McEwen, W. J. (1978). A study of the relationship between pantomime symbolism and pantomime recognition in aphasia. *Folia Phoniatrica, 30,* 286–292.

Duffy, J. M., and Ulrich, S. R. (1976). A comparison of impairments in verbal comprehension, speech, reading, and writing in adult aphasics. *Journal of Speech and Hearing Disorders, 41,* 110–119.

Duffy, J. R., and Watkins, L. B. (1984). The effect of response choice relatedness on pantomime and verbal recognition ability in aphasic patients. *Brain and Language, 21,* 291–306.

Dunlop, J. M., and Marquardt, T. P. (1977). Linguistic and articulatory aspects of single word production in apraxia of speech. *Cortex, 13,* 17–29.

Dunn, J. M., Horton, K. B., and Smith, J. O. (1968). *Peabody language development kits: Level P.* American Guidance Service (Division of Psychan Ltd., Willowdale, Ont.).

Dunn, L. M., and Smith, J. O. (1966). *Peabody language development kits: Level 2.* American Guidance Service (Division of Psychan Ltd., Willowdale, Ont.).

Dunn., L. M., and Smith, J. O. (1967). *Peabody language development kits: Level 3.* American Guidance Service (Division of Psychan Ltd., Willowdale, Ont.).

Eagleson, H. T., Vaughn, G. R., and Knudson, A. B. (1970). Hand signals for dysphasia. *Archives of Physical Medicine and Rehabilitation, 51,* 111–113.

Easterbrook, A., Brown, B. B., and Perera, K. (1982). A comparison of the speech of adult aphasic subjects in spontaneous and structured interactions. *British Journal of Disorders of Communication, 17,* 93–107.

Eisenson, J. (1949). Prognostic factors related to language rehabilitation in aphasic patients. *Journal of Speech Disorders, 14,* 262–264.

Eisenson, J. (1971). Therapeutic problems and approaches with aphasic adults. In L. E. Travis (Ed.), *Handbook of speech pathology and audiology.* New York: Appleton-Century-Crofts.

Eisenson, J. (1984). *Adult aphasia* (2nd ed.). Englewood Cliffs, NJ: Prentice-Hall.

Ellis, A. W. (1982). Spelling and writing (and reading and speaking). In A. W. Ellis (Ed.), *Normality and pathology in cognitive functions.* London: Academic Press.

Faber, M. M., and Aten, J. L. (1979). Verbal performance in aphasic patients in response to intact and altered pictorial stimuli. In R. H. Brookshire (Ed.), *Clinical aphasiology conference proceedings* (pp. 177–186). Minneapolis: BRK Publishers.

Familiar sounds. (1972). Developmental Learning Materials (Division of PMB Industries, Scarborough, Ont.).

Ferguson, J., and Boller, F. (1977). A different form of agraphia: Writing errors in patients with motor, speech and movement disorders. *Brain and Language, 4,* 382–389.

Feyereisen, P., and Seron, X. (1982). Nonverbal communication and aphasia: A review. 1. Comprehension. *Brain and Language, 16,* 191–212.

Filby, Y., Edwards, A. E., and Seacat, G. F. (1963). Word length, frequency and similarity in the discrimination behavior of aphasics. *Journal of Speech and Hearing Research, 6,* 255–261.

Fillmore, C. (1968). The case for case. In E. Bach and R. J. Harms (Eds.), *Universals in linguistic theory.* New York: Holt, Rinehart and Winston.

Fillmore, C. (1975). The case for case reopened. In P. Cole and J. Sadock (Eds.), *Syntax and semantics: Grammatical relations.* New York: Academic Press.

Flesch, R. (1951). *How to test readability.* New York: Harper & Row.

Franz, S. I. (1906). The reeducation of an aphasic. *Journal of Philosophy, Psychology and Scientific Methods, 2,* 589–597.

Franz, S. I. (1924). Studies in re-education: The aphasics. *Journal of Comparative Psychology, 4,* 349–429

Frazier, C. H., and Ingham, D. (1920). A review of the effects of gun-shot wounds of the head. *Archives of Neurology and Psychiatry, 3,* 17–40.

Freedman-Stern, R., Ulatowska, H. K., Baker, T., and Delacoste, C. (1984). Description of written language in aphasia: A case study. *Brain and Language, 22,* 181–205.

Friederici, A. D. (1981). Production and comprehension of prepositions in aphasia. *Neuropsychologia, 13,* 212–222.

Friederici, A. D., Schoenle, P. W., and Goodglass, H. (1981). Mechanisms underlying writing and speech in aphasia. *Brain and Language, 13,* 212–222.

Friedman, R. B. (1981). Preservation of orthographic knowledge in aphasia. *Brain and Language, 14,* 307–314.

Friedman, R. B., and Perlman, M. B. (1982). On the underlying causes of semantic paralexias in a patient with deep dyslexia. *Neuropsychologia, 20,* 559–568.

Fry, E. B. (1968). A readability formula that saves time. *Journal of Reading, 11,* 513–516, 575–578.

Gainotti, G., and Lemmo, M. (1976). Comprehension of symbolic gestures in aphasia. *Brain and Language, 3,* 451–460.

Gainotti, G., Micheli, G., Silveri, M. C., and Villa, G. (1983). The production of morphological and lexical opposites in aphasia. *Neuropsychologia, 21,* 693–697.

Gallagher, T. M., and Guilford, A. M. (1977). Wh-questions: Responses by aphasic patients. *Cortex, 13,* 44–54.

Gallaher, A. J., and Canter, G. J. (1982). Reading and listening comprehension in Broca's aphasia: Lexical versus syntactical errors. *Brain and Language, 17,* 183–192.

Gardiner, B. V., and Brookshire, R. H. (1972). Effects of unisensory and multisensory presentation of stimuli upon naming by aphasic subjects. *Language and Speech, 15,* 354–357.

Gardner, H. (1973). The contribution of operativity to naming in aphasic patients. *Neuropsychologia, 11,* 213–220.

Gardner, H. (1974a). The naming and recognition of written symbols in aphasic and alexic patients. *Journal of Communication Disorders, 7,* 141–154.

Gardner, H. (1974b). The naming of objects and symbols by children and aphasic patients. *Journal of Psycholinguistic Research, 3,* 133–149.

Gardner, H., Denes, G., and Zurif, E. (1975). Critical reading at the sentence level in aphasia. *Cortex, 11,* 60–72.

Gardner, H., and Winner, E. (1978). A study of repetition in aphasic patients. *Brain and Language, 6,* 168–178.

Gardner, H., and Zurif, E. (1975). Bee but not be: Oral reading of single words in aphasia and alexia. *Neuropsychologia, 13,* 181–190.

Gardner, H., and Zurif, E. (1976). Critical reading of words and phrases in aphasia. *Brain and Language, 3,* 173–190.

Gardner, H., Zurif, E. B., Berry, T., and Baker, E. (1976). Visual communication in aphasia. *Neuropsychologia, 14,* 275–292.

Gazzaniga, M. S., Glass, A. V., Sarno, M. T., and Posner, J. B. (1973). Pure word deafness and hemispheric dynamics: A case history. *Cortex, 9,* 136–143.

Geschwind, N. (1967). The varieties of naming errors. *Cortex, 3,* 97–112.

Geschwind, N., and Fusillo, M. (1966). Color naming defects in association with alexia. *Archives of Neurology, 15,* 137–146.

Geschwind, N., and Kaplan, E. (1962). A human cerebral deconnection syndrome. *Neurology, 12,* 675–685.

Gibson, J. W., Gruner, C. R., Kibler, R. J., and Kelly, F. J. (1966). A quantitative examination of differences and similarities in written and spoken languages. *Speech Monographs, 33,* 444–451.

Gleason, J. B., Goodglass, H., Green, E., Ackerman, N., and Hyde, M. R. (1975). The retrieval of syntax in Broca's aphasia. *Brain and Language, 2,* 451–471.

Gleason, J., Goodglass, H., Obler, L., Green, E., Hyde, M. R., and Weintraub, S. (1980). Narrative strategies of aphasic and normal-speaking subjects. *Journal of Speech and Hearing Research, 23,* 370–382.

Gloning, K., Trappl, R., Heiss, W-D., and Quatember, R. (1976). Prognosis and speech therapy in aphasia. In Y. Lebrun and R. Hoops (Eds.), *Recovery in aphasics.* Amsterdam: Swets & Zeitlinger BV.

Godfrey, C. M., and Douglass, E. (1959). The recovery process in aphasia. *Canadian Medical Association Journal, 80,* 618–624.

Goldberg, T., and Benjamins, D. (1982). The possible existence of phonemic reading in the presence of Broca's aphasia: A case report. *Neuropsychologia, 20,* 547–558.

Goldstein, H., and Cameron, H. (1952). New method of communication for aphasic patients. *Arizona Medicine, 8,* 1721.

Goodglass, H. (1968). Studies on the grammar of aphasics. In S. Rosenberg and J. Koplin (Eds.), *Developments in applied psycholinguistic research* (pp. 177–208). New York: Macmillan.

Goodglass, H. (1975). Phonological factors in aphasia. In R. H. Brookshire (Ed.), *Clinical aphasiology conference proceedings* (pp. 132–144). Minneapolis: BRK Publishers.

Goodglass, H. (1976). Agrammatism. In H. Whitaker and H. A. Whitaker (Eds.), *Studies in neurolinguistics* (Vol. 1, pp. 237–260). New York: Academic Press.

Goodglass, H. (1980). Disorders of naming following brain injury. *American Scientist, 68,* 647–655.

Goodglass, H., Barton, M., and Kaplan, E. (1968). Sensory modality and object-naming in aphasia. *Journal of Speech and Hearing Research, 11,* 488–496.

Goodglass, H., and Berko, J. (1960). Aphasia and inflectional morphology in English. *Journal of Speech and Hearing Research, 10,* 257–262.

Goodglass, H., Blumstein, S. E., Gleason, J. B., Hyde, M. R., Green, E., and Statlender, S. (1979). The effect of syntactic encoding on sentence comprehension in aphasia. *Brain and Language, 7,* 201–209.

Goodglass, H., Fodor, I. G., and Schulhoff, C. L. (1967). Prosodic factors in grammar—evidence from aphasia. *Journal of Speech and Hearing Research, 10,* 5–20.

Goodglass, H., Gleason, J. B., Bernholtz, N. A., and Hyde, M. R. (1972). Some linguistic structures in the speech of a Broca's aphasic. *Cortex, 8,* 191–212.

Goodglass, H., Gleason, J. B., and Hyde, M. R. (1970). Some dimensions of auditory language comprehension in aphasia. *Journal of Speech and Hearing Research, 13,* 595–606.

Goodglass, H., and Hunter, M. (1970). A linguistic comparison of speech and writing in two types of aphasia. *Communication Disorders, 3,* 28–35.

Goodglass, H., and Kaplan, E. (1963). Disturbance of gesture and pantomime in aphasia. *Brain, 86,* 703–720.

Goodglass, H., and Kaplan, E. (1972). *The assessment of aphasia and related disorders.* Philadelphia: Lea & Febiger.

Goodglass, H., and Kaplan, E. (1983). *The assessment of aphasia and related disorders* (2nd ed.). Philadelphia: Lea & Febiger.

Goodglass, H., Kaplan, E., Weintraub, S., and Ackerman, N. (1976). The "tip-of-the-tongue" phenomenon in aphasia. *Cortex, 12,* 145–153.

Goodglass, H., Klein, B., Carey, P. W., and Jones, K. J. (1966). Specific semantic word categories in aphasia. *Cortex, 2,* 74–89.

Goodglass, H., and Stuss, D. T. (1979). Naming to picture versus description in three aphasic subgroups. *Cortex, 15,* 199–211.

Green, E. (1969). Phonological and grammatical aspects of jargon in an aphasic patient: A case study. *Language and Speech, 12,* 103–118.

Green, E., and Boller, F. (1974). Features of auditory comprehension in severely impaired aphasics. *Cortex, 10,* 133–145.

Griffith, J., and Miner, L. E. (1973). *Drill materials unit.* Bell and Howell (Division of Charles E. Merrill Pub., Weston, Ont.).

Griffith, V. E. (1970). *A stroke in the family.* Baltimore: Penguin Books.

Grossman, M. (1978). The game of the name: An examination of linguistic reference after brain damage. *Brain and Language, 6,* 112–119.

Guilford, A. M., Scheurele, J., and Shirek, P. G. (1982). Manual communication skills in aphasia. *Archives of Physical Medicine and Rehabilitation, 63,* 601–604.

Gunning, R. (1968). *The technique of clear writing.* New York: McGraw-Hill.

Gurland, G., Chwat, S., and Gerber-Wollner, S. (1982). Establishing a communication profile in adult aphasia: Analysis of communicative acts and conversational sequences. In R. H. Brookshire (Ed.), *Clinical aphasiology conference proceedings.* Minneapolis: BRK Publishers.

Hagen, C. (1973). Communication abilities in hemiplegia: Effect of speech therapy. *Archives of Physical Medicine and Rehabilitation, 54,* 454–463.

Hain, R., and Lainer, H. (1977). *Language rehabilitation program: Level 1.* Teaching Resources Corp. (Division of Ginn & Company, Scarborough, Ont.).

Hain, R., and Lanier, H. (1980). *Language rehabilitation program: Level 2.* Teaching Resources Corp. (Division of Ginn & Company, Scarborough, Ont.).

Hardison, D., Marquardt, T. P., and Peterson, H. A. (1977). Effects of selected linguistic variables on apraxia of speech. *Journal of Speech and Hearing Research, 20,* 334–343.

Hatfield, F. M., Howard, D., Barber, J., Jones, C., and Morton, J. (1977). Object naming in aphasics—the lack of effect of context or realism. *Neuropsychologia, 15,* 717–727.

Hécaen, H., and Albert, M. L. (1978). *Human Neuropsychology* (pp. 58-67). New York: John Wiley and Sons.

Hécaen, H., and Kremin, H. (1976). Neurolinguistic research on reading disorders resulting from left hemisphere lesions: Aphasia and "pure" alexias. In H. Whitaker and H. A. Whitaker (Eds.), *Studies in neurolinguistics: Vol. 2* (pp. 269–329). New York: Academic Press.

Helm, N. A., and Barresi, B. (1980). Voluntary control of involuntary utterances: A treatment approach for severe aphasia. In R. H. Brookshire (Ed.), *Clinical aphasiology conference proceedings* (pp. 308–315). Minneapolis: BRK Publishers.

Helm, N., and Benson, D. F. (1978). *Visual action therapy for global aphasia.*

Paper presented at the 16th annual meeting of the Academy of Aphasia, Chicago.

Helm-Estabrooks, N. (1981). *Helm elicited language program for syntax stimulation*. Austin: Exceptional Resources, Inc.

Helm-Estabrooks, N., Fitzpatrick, P. M., and Barresi, B. (1982). Visual action therapy for global aphasia. *Journal of Speech and Hearing Disorders, 47,* 385–389.

Helmick, J. W., and Wipplingler, M. (1975). Effects of stimulus repetition on the naming behaviour of an aphasic adult: A clinical report. *Journal of Communication Disorders, 8,* 23–29.

Henri, B. (1973). *A longitudinal investigation of patterns of language recovery in eight aphasic patients.* Unpublished doctoral dissertation, Northwestern University, Evanston, IL.

Hier, D. B., and Mohr, J. P. (1977). Incongruous oral and written naming. *Brain and Language, 4,* 115–126.

Holland, A. L. (1975). The effectiveness of treatment in aphasia. In R. H. Brookshire (Ed.), *Clinical aphasiology conference proceedings.* Minneapolis: BRK Publishers.

Holland, A. L. (1980). *Communicative abilities in daily living.* Baltimore: University Park Press.

Holland, A. L. (1982). Observing functional communication of aphasic adults. *Journal of Speech and Hearing Disorders, 17,* 50–56.

Holland, A., Bartlett, C. L., Fromm, D., Pashek, G., Stein, D., and Swindell, C. (October, 1982). *Rapid recovery of language following cerebral infarction: A case study.* Paper presented at the 20th annual meeting of the Academy of Aphasia, Lake Mohonk, NY.

Hoodin, R. B., and Thompson, C. K. (1983). Facilitation of verbal labeling in adult aphasia by gestural, verbal, or verbal plus gestural training (Abstract). In R. H. Brookshire (Ed.), *Clinical aphasiology conference proceedings.* Minneapolis: BRK Publishers.

Howes, D., and Geschwind, N. (1964). Quantitative studies of aphasic language. In D. McK. Rioch and E. A. Weinstein (Eds.), *Disorders of communication.* Baltimore: Williams & Wilkins.

Itoh, M., Sasanuma, S., and Ushijima, T. (1979). Velar movements during speech in a patient with apraxia of speech. *Brain and Language, 7,* 227–239.

Jenkins, J., Jiménez-Pabón, E., Shaw, R., and Sefer, J. (1975). *Schuell's aphasia in adults* (2nd ed.). New York: Harper & Row.

Johns, D., and Darley, F. L. (1970). Phonemic variability in apraxia of speech. *Journal of Speech and Hearing Research, 13,* 556–583.

Kaplan, E., and Goodglass, H. (1981). Aphasia—related disorders. In M. T. Sarno (Ed.), *Acquired aphasia.* New York: Academic Press.

Kapur, N., and Perl, N. T. (1978). Recognition reading in paralexia. *Cortex, 14,* 439–443.

Kearns, K. P. (1980). The application of phonological process analysis to adult neuropathologies. In R. H. Brookshire (Ed.), *Clinical aphasiology conference proceedings* (pp. 187–195). Minneapolis: BRK Publishers.

Keenan, J. S. (1975). *A procedure manual in speech pathology with brain-damaged adults.* Danville, IL: Interstate Press.

Keenan, J. S., and Brassell, E. G. (1972). Comparison of minimally dysphasic and minimally educated subjects in a sentence writing task. *Cortex, 8,* 93–105.

Kellar, L. A. (1978). *Stress and syntax in aphasia.* Paper presented at the Academy of Aphasia, Chicago.

Kertesz, A., and Poole, E. (1974). The aphasia quotient: The taxonomic approach to measurement of aphasic disability. *Canadian Journal of Neurological Sciences, 1,* 7–16.

Kimura, D. (1982). Left-hemisphere control of oral and brachial movements and their relation to communication. *Philosophy Transactions of the Royal Society of London, 25; 298* (1089), 135–149.

Kinsbourne, M., and Rosenfield, D. B. (1974). Agraphia selective for written spelling. *Brain and Language, 1,* 215–225.

Kirshner, H. S., and Webb, W. G. (1981). Selective involvement of the auditory-verbal modality in an acquired communication disorder: Benefit from sign language therapy. *Brain and Language, 13,* 161–170.

Kohn, S. E. (1984). The nature of phonological disorder in conduction aphasia. *Brain and Language, 23,* 97–115.

Kreindler, A., Fradis, A., and Mihailescu, L. (1983). Quantitative studies on speech characteristics of aphasics: A statistical approach to vocabulary. *Human Neurobiology, 2,* 171–176.

Kučera, H., and Francis, W. N. (1967). *Computational analysis of present day English.* Providence, RI: Brown University Press.

Kurtzke, J. F. (1976). An introduction to the epidemiology of cerebrovascular disease. In P. Scheinberg (Ed.), *Cerebrovascular diseases: Tenth Princeton conference.* New York: Raven Press.

Langmore, S. E., and Canter, G. J. (1983). Written spelling deficit of Broca's aphasics. *Brain and Language, 18,* 293–314.

LaPointe, L. L. (1977). Base-10 programmed stimulation: Task specification, scoring, and plotting performance in aphasia therapy. *Journal of Speech and Hearing Disorders, 42,* 90–105.

LaPointe, L. L. (1983). Aphasia intervention with adults: historical, present, and future approaches. In J. Miller, D. E. Yoder, R. Schiefelbusch (Eds.), *Contemporary issues in language intervention* (ASHA Reports 12). Rockville, MD: The American Speech-Language-Hearing Association.

Lecours, A. R., L'hermitte, F., and Bryans, B. (1983). *Aphasiology.* London: Baillière Tindall.

Lee, J. (1980). A note on the comparison of group means based on repeated measurements of the same subject. *Journal of Chronic Diseases, 33,* 673–675.

Leischner, A. (1983). Side differences in writing to dictation of aphasics with agraphia: A graphic disconnection. *Brain and Language, 18,* 1–19.

Lemme, M. L., Hedberg, N. L., and Bottenberg, D. E. (1984). Cohesion in narratives of aphasic adults. In R. H. Brookshire (Ed.), *Clinical aphasiology conference proceedings.* Minneapolis: BRK Publishers.

Lesser, R. (1974). Verbal comprehension in aphasia: An English version of three Italian tests. *Cortex, 10,* 247–263.

Lesser, R. (1978). *Linguistic investigations of aphasia.* London: Arnold.

Levy, C. B., and Taylor, O. L. (1968). *Transformational complexity and comprehension in adult aphasics.* Paper presented at the annual convention of the American Speech-Language-Hearing Association, Denver.

L'hermitte, F., Dérouesné, J., and Lecours, A. R. (1971). Contribution à l'étude des troubles sémantiques dans l'aphasie. *Révue Neurologique, 125,* 81-101.

Li, E. C., and Canter, G. J. (1983). Phonemic cuing: An investigation of subject variables. In R. H. Brookshire (Ed.), *Clinicial aphasiology conference proceedings.* Minneapolis: BRK Publishers.

Linebaugh, C., Kryzer, K., Oden, S., and Myers, P. (1982). Reapportionment of communicative burden in aphasia: A study of narrative interactions. In R. H. Brookshire (Ed.), *Clinical aphasiology conference proceedings*. Minneapolis: BRK Publishers.

Locke, J. L., and Deck, J. W. (1982). The processing of printed language by aphasic adults: Some phonological and syntactic effects. *Journal of Speech and Hearing Research, 25,* 314–319.

Love, R. J., and Webb, W. G. (1977). The efficacy of cueing techniques in Broca's aphasia. *Journal of Speech and Hearing Disorders, 42,* 170–178.

Ludlow, C. L. (1973). *The recovery of syntax in aphasia: An analysis of syntactic structures used in connected speech during the initial recovery period.* Unpublished doctoral dissertation, New York University.

Luria, A. R. (1966). *Higher cortical functions in man.* New York: Basic Books.

Luria, A. R. (1980). *Higher cortical functions in man* (2nd ed.). New York: Basic Books.

MacKenzie, C. (1982). Aphasic articulatory defect and aphasic phonological defect. *British Journal of Disorders of Communication, 17,* 27–46.

Marcie, P., and Hécaen, H. (1979). Agraphia: Writing disorders associated with unilateral cortical lesions. In K. M. Heilman and E. Valenstein (Eds.), *Clinical Neuropsychology.* New York: Oxford University Press.

Margolin, D. I. (1984). The neuropsychology of writing and spelling: Semantic phonological, motor and perceptual processes. *Quarterly Journal of Experimental Psychology, 36A,* 459–489.

Margolin, D. I., and Binder, L. (1984). Multiple component agraphia in a patient with atypical cerebral dominance: An error analysis. *Brain and Language, 22,* 26–40.

Marks, M., Taylor, M., and Rusk, H. (1957). Rehabilitation of the aphasic patient: A survey of three years' experience in a rehabilitation setting. *Archives of Physical Medicine and Rehabilitation, 38,* 219–226.

Marshall, J. C., and Newcombe, F. (1966). Syntactic and semantic errors in paralexia. *Neuropsychologia, 4,* 169–176.

Marshall, J. C., and Newcombe, F. (1973). Patterns of paralexia: A psycholinguistic approach. *Journal of Psycholinguistic Research, 2,* 175–199.

Marshall, R. C. (1976). Word retrieval behaviour of aphasic adults. *Journal of Speech and Hearing Disorders, 41,* 444–451.

Marshall, R. C., and Stevenson, S. A. (1977). Pure word deafness: Fact or fiction. In R. H. Brookshire (Ed.), *Clinical aphasiology conference proceedings* (pp. 248–256). Minneapolis: BRK Publishers.

Martin, A. D. (1973). *Some objections to the term "apraxia of speech."* Paper presented to the Third Clinical Aphasiology Conference, Albuquerque.

Martin, A. D., Kornberg, S., Hoffnung, A., and Gerstman, L. (1978). The effect of grammatic context on repetition by aphasic adults. In R. H. Brookshire (Ed.), *Clinical aphasiology conference proceedings* (pp. 236–246). Minneapolis: BRK Publishers.

Martin, A. D., and Rigrodsky, S. (1974a). An investigation of phonological impairment in aphasia, Part 1. *Cortex, 10,* 317–328.

Martin, A. D., and Rigrodsky, S. (1974b). An investigation of phonological impairment in aphasia, Part 2: Distinctive feature analysis of phonetic commutation errors in aphasia. *Cortex, 10,* 329–346.

Martin, R., Caramazza, A., and Berndt, R. S. (1982). *Oral reading and writing in agrammatic aphasics.* Paper presented at the Academy of Aphasia, Lake Mohonk, NY.

McLaughlin, G. (1969). SMOG Grading—A new readability formula. *Journal of Reading, 12,* 639–646.

Medlin, W. L. (1975). *Word making cards.* Salt Lake City: Word Making Productions.

Mercaitis, P. A., and Duffy, J. R. (1984). Verbal response time and intersyllable interval in the imitative speech of non-brain-injured aphasic and apraxic adults (Abstract). In R. H. Brookshire (Ed.), *Clinical aphasiology conference proceedings.* Minneapolis: BRK Publishers.

Mills, C. K. (1904). Treatment of aphasia by training. *Journal of American Medical Association, 43,* 1940–1949.

Mills, R. H., Knox, A. W., Juola, J. F., and Salmon, S. J. (1979). Cognitive loci of impairments in picture naming by aphasic subjects. *Journal of Speech and Hearing Research, 22,* 73–87.

Monoi, H., Fukusako, Y., Itoh, M., and Sasanuma, S. (1983). Speech sound errors in patients with conduction and Broca's aphasia. *Brain and Language, 20,* 175–194.

Moody, E. J. (1982). Sign language acquisition by a global aphasic. *The Journal of Nervous and Mental Disease, 170,* 113–116.

Myerson, R., and Goodglass, H. (1972). Transformational grammars of three agrammatic patients. *Language and Speech, 15,* 40–50.

Netsu, R., and Marquardt, T. P. (1984). Pantomime in aphasia: Effects of stimulus characteristics. *Journal of Communication Disorders, 17,* 37–46.

Oldfield, R., and Wingfield, A. (1965). Response latencies in naming objects. *Quarterly Journal of Experimental Psychology, 17,* 273–281.

Parisi, P., and Pizzamiglio, L. (1970). Syntactic comprehension in aphasia. *Cortex, 6,* 204–215.

Pashek, G. V., and Brookshire, R. H. (1980). Effects of rate of speech and linguistic stress on auditory paragraph comprehension of aphasic individuals. In R. H. Brookshire (Ed.), *Clinical aphasiology conference proceedings* (pp. 64–65, Abstract). Minneapolis: BRK Publishers.

Patterson, K. E., and Marcel, A. J. (1977). Aphasia, dyslexia, and phonological coding of written words. *Quarterly Journal of Experimental Psychology, 29,* 307–318.

Peacher, W. G. (1946). Speech disorders in World War II: V. Organization of a speech clinic in an army hospital. *Journal of Speech Disorders, 11,* 233–239.

Pease, D. M., and Goodglass, H. (1978). The effects of cuing on picture naming in aphasia. *Cortex, 14,* 178–189.

Peterson, L. N., and Kirshner, H. S. (1981). Gestural impairment and gestural ability in aphasia: A review. *Brain and Language, 14,* 580–594.

Piehler, M. F., and Holland, A. L. (1984). Cohesion in aphasic language. In R. H. Brookshire (Ed.), *Clinical aphasiology conference proceedings.* Minneapolis: BRK Publishers.

Pierce, R. S. (1979). A study of sentence comprehension of aphasic subjects. In R. H. Brookshire (Ed.), *Clinical aphasiology conference proceedings* (pp. 213–226). Minneapolis: BRK Publishers.

Pierce, R. S. (1981). Cuing efficiency in aphasia: A case study. *Aphasia Apraxia Agnosia, 3,* 13–26.

Podraza, B. L., and Darley, F. L. (1977). Effect of auditory prestimulation on naming in aphasia. *Journal of Speech and Hearing Research, 20,* 669–683.

Pöeck, K. (1982). *Modern methods of aphasia therapy.* Paper presented at the seventh annual meeting of the Japanese CVD Society, Hirosaki, Japan.

Poizner, H., Bellugi, U., and Iraqui, V. (1984). Apraxia and aphasia for a visual-gestural language. *American Journal of Physiology, 246,* R868–83.

Porch, B. E. (1967). *Porch index of communicative ability.* Palo Alto, CA: Consulting Psychologists Press.

Porch, B. E. (1971). *Porch index of communicative ability* (rev. ed.). Palo Alto, CA: Consulting Psychologists Press.

Porch, B. E. (1981). *Porch index of communicative ability* (Vol. 2, 3rd ed.). Palo Alto, CA: Consulting Psychologists Press.

Prins, R. S., Snow, C. E., and Wagenaar, E. (1978). Recovery from aphasia: Spontaneous speech versus language comprehension. *Brain and Language, 6,* 192–211.

Rao, P. R., and Horner, J. (1978). Gesture as deblocking modality in a severe aphasic patient. In R. H. Brookshire (Ed.), *Clinical aphasiology conference proceedings.* Minneapolis: BRK Publishers.

Raven, J. (1956). *Coloured progressive matrices: Sets A, A$_B$, B.* (Revised Order). London: Lewis and Company Limited.

Richardson, J. (1975). The effect of word imageability in acquired dyslexia. *Neuropsychologia, 13,* 281–288.

Riese, W. (1947). The early history of aphasia. *Bulletin of the History of Medicine, 23,* 322–334.

Rochford, G., and Williams, M. (1965). Studies in the development and breakdown of the use of names. *Journal of Neurosurgery and Psychiatry, 28,* 407–412.

Roeltgen, D. P., and Heilman, K. M. (1983). Apractic agraphia in a patient with normal praxis. *Brain and Language, 18,* 35–46.

Roeltgen, D. P., and Heilman, K. M. (1984). Lexical agraphia: Further support for the two-system hypothesis of linguistic agraphia. *Brain, 107,* 811–827.

Roeltgen, D. P., Rothi, L. J., and Heilman, K. M. (1982). Semantic agraphia (abstract). *Annals of Neurology, 12,* 95.

Roeltgen, D. P., Sevush, S., and Heilman, K. M. (1983). Phonological agraphia: Writing by the lexical semantic route. *Neurology, 33,* 755–765.

Rosenbek, J. C., Lemme, M. L., Ahern, M. B., Harris, E. H., and Wertz, R. T. (1973). A treatment for apraxia of speech in adults. *Journal of Speech and Hearing Disorders, 38,* 462–472.

Rothi, L. J., and Heilman, K. M. (1981). Alexia and agraphia with spared spelling letter recognition abilities. *Brain and Language, 12,* 1–13.

Rothi, L. J., McFarling, D., and Heilman, K. M. (1982).Conduction aphasia, syntactic alexia, and the anatomy of syntactic comprehension. *Archives of Neurology, 39,* 272–275.

Saffran, E. M., and Marin, O. S. (1977). Reading without phonology: Evidence from aphasia. *Quarterly Journal of Experimental Psychology, 29,* 515–525.

Saffran, E. M., Marin, O. S., and Yeni-Komshian, G. H. (1976). An analysis of speech perception in word deafness. *Brain and Language, 3,* 209–228.

Saffran, E. M., Schwartz, M. F., and Marin, O. S. (1980). The word order problem in agrammatism: II. Production. *Brain and Language, 10,* 263–280.

Salvatore, A., Trunzo, M., Holtzapple, P., and Graham, L. (1983). Investigation of the sentence hierarchy of the Helm Elicited Language Program for Syntax Stimulation. In R. H. Brookshire (Ed.), *Clinical aphasiology conference proceedings.* Minneapolis: BRK Publishers.

Samuels, J. A., and Benson, D. F. (1979). Some aspects of language comprehension in anterior aphasia. *Brain and Language, 8,* 275–286.

Sanders, S. B., Davis, G. A., and Hubler, V. (1979). A study of the interdependence of word retrieval and repetition in conduction aphasia. In R. H. Brookshire (Ed.), *Clinical aphasiology conference proceedings* (pp. 270–277). Minneapolis: BRK Publishers.

Sands, E. S., Sarno, M. T., and Shankweiler, D. P. (1969). Long-term assessment of language function in aphasia due to stroke. *Archives of Physical Medicine, 50,* 202–206.

Sarno, M. T., and Levita, E. (1971). Natural course of recovery in severe aphasia. *Archives of Physical Medicine and Rehabilitation, 52*, 175–178.

Sarno, M. T., Silverman, M., and Sands, E. S. (1970). Speech therapy and language recovery in severe aphasia. *Journal of Speech and Hearing Research, 13*, 607–623.

Sartori, G., Bruno, S., Serena, M., and Bardin, P. (1984). Deep dyslexia in a patient with crossed aphasia. *European Neurology, 23*, 95–99.

Scargill, M. H. (1954). Modern linguistics and recovery from aphasia. *Journal of Speech and Hearing Disorders, 19*, 507–514.

Schlanger, P. H., and Freemann, R. (1979). Pantomime therapy with aphasics. *Aphasia-Apraxia-Agnosia, 1*, 34–39.

Schlanger, P. H., and Schlanger, B. B. (1970). Adapting role playing activities with aphasic patients. *Journal of Speech and Hearing Disorders, 35*, 229–235.

Schuell, H. M., and Jenkins, J. J. (1961). Reduction of vocabulary in aphasia. *Brain, 84*, 243–261.

Schuell, H., Jenkins, J. J., and Jiménez-Pabón, E. (1964). *Aphasia in adults: Diagnosis, prognosis, and treatment.* New York: Harper & Row.

Schuell, H. M., Jenkins, J. J., and Landis, L. (1961). Relationship between auditory comprehension and word frequency in aphasia. *Journal of Speech and Hearing Research, 4*, 30–36.

Searle, J. R. (1969). *Speech acts.* London: Cambridge University Press.

Sefer, J. W. (1973). A case study demonstrating the value of aphasia therapy. *British Journal of Disorders of Communication, 8*, 99–104.

Seron, X., Deloche, G., Bastard, V., Chassin, G., and Hermand, N. (1979a). Word-finding difficulties and learning transfer in aphasic patients. *Cortex, 15*, 149–155.

Seron, X., van der Kaa, M. A., Remitz, A., and van der Linden, M. (1979b). Pantomime interpretation and aphasia. *Neuropsychologia, 17*, 661–668.

Shallice, T. (1981). Phonological agraphia and the lexical route in writing. *Brain, 104*, 413–429.

Shallice, T., and Coughlan, A. K. (1980). Modality specific word comprehension deficits in deep dyslexia. *Journal of Neurology, Neurosurgery, and Psychiatry, 43*, 866–872.

Shallice, T., and Warrington, E. (1975). Word recognition in a phonemic dyslexic patient. *Quarterly Journal of Experimental Psychology, 27*, 515–525.

Shankweiler, D., and Harris, K. S. (1966). An experimental approach to the problem of articulation in aphasia. *Cortex, 2*, 277–292.

Shewan, C. M. (Undated). *Easing the communication load with the aphasic patient.* Unpublished manuscript. The University of Western Ontario, London, Ontario.

Shewan, C. M. (1976a). Error patterns in auditory comprehension of adult aphasics. *Cortex, 12*, 325–336.

Shewan, C. M. (1976b). Facilitating sentence formulation: A case study. *Journal of Communication Disorders, 9*, 191–197.

Shewan, C. M. (1977). *Procedures manual for speech and language training: Language-Oriented Therapy (LOT).* Unpublished manuscript. The University of Western Ontario, London, Ontario.

Shewan, C. M. (1979). *Auditory Comprehension Test for Sentences (ACTS).* Chicago: Biolinguistics Clinical Institutes.

Shewan, C. M. (1980a). Phonological processing in Broca's aphasics. *Brain and Language, 10*, 71–88.

Shewan, C. M. (1980b). Verbal dyspraxia and its treatment. *Human Com-*

munication, 5, 3–12.

Shewan, C. M. (1982). To hear is not to understand: Auditory processing deficits and factors influencing performance in aphasic individuals. In N. J. Lass (Ed.), *Speech and language: Advances in basic research and practice* (Vol. 7, pp. 1–70). New York: Academic Press.

Shewan, C. M. (1985). The history and efficacy of aphasia treatment. In R. Chapey (Ed.), *Language intervention strategies in adult aphasia* (2nd ed.). Baltimore: Williams & Wilkins.

Shewan, C. M., and Cameron, H. (1984). Communication and related problems as perceived by aphasic individuals and their spouses. *Journal of Communication Disorders, 17,* 175–187.

Shewan, C. M., and Canter, G. J. (1971). Effects of vocabulary, syntax, and sentence length on auditory comprehension of aphasic patients. *Cortex, 7,* 209–226.

Shewan, C. M., and Henderson, V. L. (1984). *Analysis of spontaneous language communication in the older normal population.* Unpublished manuscript, University of Western Ontario, London, Canada.

Shewan, C. M., and Kertesz, A. (1983). *Language therapy and recovery from aphasia.* Final project report. DM324 Grant, Ontario Ministry of Health.

Shewan, C. M., and Kertesz, A. (1984). Effects of speech and language treatment on recovery from aphasia. *Brain and Language, 23,* 272–299.

Shewan, C. M., Leeper, H. A., Jr., and Booth, J. C. (1984). An analysis of voice onset time (VOT) in aphasic and normal subjects. In J. C. Rosenbek, M. R. McNeil, and A. E. Aronson (Eds.), *Apraxia of Speech.* San Diego: College-Hill Press.

Simmons, N. N., and Zorthian, A. (1979). Use of symbolic gestures in a case of fluent aphasia. In R. H. Brookshire (Ed.), *Clinical aphasiology conference proceedings.* Minneapolis: BRK Publishers.

Skelly, M. (1975). Re-thinking stroke: Aphasic patients talk back. *American Journal of Nursing, 75,* 1140–1142.

Skelly, M. (1979). *Amer-Ind gestural code.* New York: Elsevier.

Skelly, M., Schinsky, L., Smith, R. W., Donaldson, R. C., and Griffin, J. M. (1975). American Indian Sign: A gestural communication system for the speechless. *Archives of Physical Medicine and Rehabilitation, 56,* 156–160.

Skelly, M., Schinsky, L., Smith, R. W., and Fust, R. S. (1974). American Indian Sign (Amer-Ind) as a facilitator of verbalization for the oral verbal apraxic. *Journal of Speech and Hearing Disorders, 39,* 446–456.

Smith, A., Champoux, R., Leri, J., London, R., and Muraski, A. (1972). *Diagnosis, intelligence and rehabilitation of chronic aphasics.* University of Michigan, Department of Physical Medicine and Rehabilitation. (Social and Rehabilitation Service, Grant No. 14–P–55198/5–01).

Spache, G. D. (1978). *Good reading for poor readers.* Champaign, IL: Garrad.

Sparks, R. W. (1981). Melodic intonation therapy. In R. Chapey (Ed.), *Language intervention strategies in adult aphasia.* Baltimore: Williams & Wilkins.

Sparks, R., Helm, N., and Albert, M. (1974). Aphasia rehabilitation resulting from Melodic Intonation Therapy. *Cortex, 10,* 303–316.

Sparks, R., and Holland, A. (1976). Method: Melodic Intonation Therapy. *Journal of Speech and Hearing Disorders, 41,* 287–297.

Spreen, O., and Schulz, R. (1966). Parameters of abstraction, meaningfulness, and pronunciability for 329 nouns. *Journal of Verbal Learning and Verbal Behavior, 5,* 459–468.

Stachowiak, F. J., Huber, W., Pöeck, K., and Kerschensteiner, M. (1977). Text comprehension in aphasia. *Brain and Language, 4*, 177–195.

Stachowiak, F., and Pöeck, K. (1976). Functional disconnection in pure alexia and colour naming deficit demonstrated by facilitation methods. *Brain and Language, 3*, 135–143.

Staller, J., Buchanan, D., Singer, M., Lappin, J., and Webb, W. (1978). Alexia without agraphia: An experimental case study. *Brain and Language, 5*, 378–387.

Stevens, E., and Glaser, L. (1983). Multiple input phoneme therapy: An approach to severe apraxia and expressive aphasia. In R. H. Brookshire (Ed.), *Clinical aphasiology conference proceedings.* Minneapolis: BRK Publishers.

Stoicheff, M. L. (1960). Motivating instructions and language performance of dysphasic subjects. *Journal of Speech and Hearing Research, 3*, 75–85.

Taylor, M. L., and Marks, M. M. (1959). *Aphasia rehabilitation and therapy kit.* Scarborough, Ont.: McGraw-Hill Ryerson.

Thorndike, E. L., and Lorge, I. (1944). *The teacher's word book of 30,000 words.* Teachers College, Columbia University, New York.

Tillman, D., and Gerstman, L. J. (1977). Clustering by aphasics in free recall. *Brain and Language, 4*, 355–364.

Tonkovich, J. D., and Marquardt, T. P. (1977). The effects of stress and melodic intonation on apraxia of speech. In R. H. Brookshire (Ed.), *Clinical aphasiology conference proceedings.* Minneapolis: BRK Publishers.

Trost, J. E. (1970). *A descriptive study of verbal apraxia in patients with Broca's aphasia.* Unpublished doctoral dissertation, Northwestern University, Evanston, IL.

Trost, J. E., and Canter, G. J. (1974). Apraxia of speech in patients with Broca's aphasia: A study of phoneme production accuracy and error patterns. *Brain and Language, 1*, 63–79.

Ulatowska, H. K., Baker, T., and Freedman-Stern, R. (1979). Disruption of written language in aphasia. In H. Whitaker and H. A. Whitaker (Eds.), *Studies in neurolinguistics* (Vol. 4, pp. 241–268). New York: Academic Press.

Ulatowska, H. K., Doyel, A. W., Stern, R. F., and Macaluso-Haynes, S. (1983a). Production of procedural discourse in aphasia. *Brain and Language, 18*, 315–341.

Ulatowska, H. K., Freedman-Stern, R., Doyel, A. W., Macaluso-Haynes, S., and North, A. J. (1983b). Production of narrative discourse in aphasia. *Brain and Language, 19*, 317–334.

Ulatowska, H., Macaluso-Haynes, S., and North, A. J. (1980). Production of narrative and procedural discourse in aphasia. In R. H. Brookshire (Ed.), *Clinical aphasiology conference proceedings* (pp. 17–27). Minneapolis: BRK Publishers.

Ulatowska, H. K., North, A. J., and Macaluso-Haynes, S. (1981). Production of narrative and procedural discourse in aphasia. *Brain and Language, 13*, 345–371.

Van Demark, A. A., Lemmer, E. C. J., and Drake, M. L. (1982). Measurement of reading comprehension in aphasia with the RCBA. *Journal of Speech and Hearing Disorders, 47*, 288–291.

Varney, N. R. (1978). Linguistic correlates of pantomime recognition in aphasic patients. *Journal of Neurology, Neurosurgery, and Psychiatry, 41*, 564–568.

Varney, N. R. (1981). Letter recognition and visual form discrimination in aphasic alexia. *Neuropsychologia, 19*, 795–800.

Varney, N. R. (1982). Pantomime recognition defect in aphasia: Implications for the concept of asymbolia. *Brain and Language, 15,* 32–39.

Varney, N. R., and Benton, A. L. (1982). Qualitative aspects of pantomime recognition defect in aphasia. *Brain and Cognition, 1,* 132–139.

Vignolo, L. A. (1964). Evolution of aphasia and language rehabilitation: A retrospective exploratory study. *Cortex, 1,* 344–367.

Vincent, F. M., Sadowsky, C. H., Saunders, R. L., and Reeves, A. G. (1977). Alexia without agraphia, hemianopia, or color-naming defect: A disconnection syndrome. *Neurology, 27,* 689–691.

von Stockert, R. T. (1972). Recognition of syntactic structure in aphasic patients. *Cortex, 8,* 323–334.

von Stockert, R. T., and Bader, L. (1976). Some relations of grammar and lexicon in aphasia. *Cortex, 12,* 49–60.

Wales, R., and Kinsella, G. (1981). Syntactic effects in sentence completion by Broca's aphasics. *Brain and Language, 13,* 301–307.

Wapner, W., and Gardner, H. (1979). A study of spelling in aphasia. *Brain and Language, 7,* 363–374.

Wapner, W., and Gardner, H. (1981). Profiles of symbol-reading skills in organic patients. *Brain and Language, 12,* 303–312.

Webb, W. G., and Love, R. J. (1983). Reading problems in chronic aphasia. *Journal of Speech and Hearing Disorders, 48,* 164–170.

Weidner, W. E., and Jinks, A. F. G. (1983). The effects of single versus combined cue presentations on picture naming by aphasic adults. *Journal of Communication Disorders, 16,* 111–121.

Weisenburg, T., and McBride, K. E. (1935). *Aphasia.* New York: Hafner Publishing Company.

Wepman, J. M. (1951). *Recovery from aphasia.* New York: The Ronald Press Company.

Wepman, J. M. (1953). A conceptual model for the processes involved in recovery from aphasia. *Journal of Speech and Hearing Disorders, 18,* 4–13.

Wepman, J. M. (1972). Aphasia therapy: A new look. *Journal of Speech and Hearing Disorders, 37,* 203–214.

Wepman, J., Bock, R., Jones, L. V., and Van Pelt, D. (1956). Psycholinguistic study of aphasia: A revision of the concept of anomia. *Journal of Speech and Hearing Disorders, 21,* 468–477.

Wertz, R. T., Collins, M., Weiss, D., Brookshire, R. H., Friden, T., Kurtzke, J. F., and Pierce, J. (1978). *Preliminary report on a comparison of individual and group treatment.* Paper presented at the annual meeting of the American Association for the Advancement of Science, Washington, DC.

Wertz, R. T., Collins, M. J., Weiss, D., Kurtzke, J. F., Frident, T., Brookshire, R. H., Pierce, J. Holtzapple, P., Hubbard, D. J., Porch, B. E., West, J. A., Davis, L., Matovitch, V., Morley, G. K., and Resurrecion, E. (1981). Veterans Administration cooperative study on aphasia: A comparison of individual and group treatment. *Journal of Speech and Hearing Research, 24,* 580–594.

Whitehouse, P., Caramazza, A., and Zurif, E. (1978). Naming in aphasia: Interacting effects of form and function. *Brain and Language, 6,* 63–74.

Whitney, J. L. (1975). *Developing aphasics' use of compensatory strategies.* Paper presented at the annual convention of the American Speech and Hearing Association, Washington, DC.

Whurr, R. (1983). *Deficits or retained areas—which to treat in aphasia?* Unpublished manuscript. Poster session presented at the annual convention of the American Speech-Language-Hearing Association, Cincinnati.

Wiegel-Crump, C., and Koenigsknecht, R. A. (1973). Tapping the lexical store of the adult aphasic: Analysis of the improvement made in word retrieval skills. *Cortex, 9,* 411–418.

Williams, M., and Owens, G. (1977). Word vs. picture recognition in amnesic and aphasic patients. *Neuropsychologia, 15,* 351–354.

Williams, S. E. (1983). Factors influencing naming performance in aphasia: A review of the literature. *Journal of Communication Disorders, 16,* 357–372.

Williams, S. E. (1984). Influence of written form on reading comprehension in aphasia. *Journal of Communication Disorders, 17,* 165–174.

Williams, S. E., and Canter, G. J. (1982). The influence of situational context on naming performance in aphasia syndromes. *Brain and Language, 17,* 92–106.

Wingfield, A. (1968). Effects of frequency on identification and naming of objects. *American Journal of Psychology, 81,* 226–234.

Wyke, M., and Holgate, D. (1973). Colour-naming defects in dysphasic patients: A qualitative analysis. *Neuropsychologia, 11,* 451–461.

Yamadori, A., and Albert, M. L. (1973). Word category aphasia. *Cortex, 9,* 112–125.

Zatorski, R. J., and Lesser, R. (1981). The lexicon and sentence generation in aphasia. *Brain and Language, 13,* 185–190.

Zurif, E. B., and Caramazza, A. (1976). Psycholinguistic structures in aphasia. In H. Whitaker and H. A. Whitaker (Eds.), *Studies in neurolinguistics* (Vol. 1). New York: Academic Press.

Zurif, E. B., Caramazza, A., and Myerson, R. (1972). Grammatical judgments of agrammatic aphasics. *Neuropsychologia, 10,* 405–417.

Zurif, E. B., Caramazza, A., Myerson, R., and Galvin, J. (1974). Semantic feature representations for normal and aphasic language. *Brain and Language, 1,* 167–187.

Zurif, E. B., Green, E., Caramazza, A., and Goodenough, C. (1976). Grammatical intuitions of aphasic patients: Sensitivity to functors. *Cortex, 12,* 183–186.

AUTHOR INDEX

SUBJECT INDEX

Abstraction
 in stimuli, 169, 186–187
 in words, 78, 92, 160, 165, 167,
  193, 212, 220
Age of subjects, 245, 246, 248, 249
Agnosia, 36
 auditory nonverbal, 36
 auditory verbal, 36
 visual, 81
Agrammatism in Broca's
  Aphasia, 7, 154, 177, 179,
  208, 213
Agraphia (see also *Graphic
  expression*), 79–80, 208–214,
  219–200
 with alexia, 79, 208, 210
 alexia without, 79–80
 aphasia and, 208
 apractic agraphia, 208
 callosal dysgraphia, 209
 deep agraphia, 212
 efferent motor agraphia, 209–210
 frontal agraphia, 208
 lexical/semantic agraphia, 208,
  212, 219
 motor and linguistic agraphia, 208
 nonaphasic agraphia, 213
 nondominant agraphia, 208
 paragraphia, 213
 parietal-temporal agraphia, 208
 phonological/nonlexical agraphia,
  208, 211–213, 220
 pure agraphia, 220
 spatial agraphia, 214
 transitional agraphia, 211
Alexia/Dyslexia (see also *Visual
  processing*), 79–81, 86, 151–152,
  165–168, 190–192
 with agraphia, 80, 167, 210
 without agraphia, 79–80, 81

central alexia, 80
deep dyslexia, 151–152, 165–166,
  168, 190–192, 212
frontal alexia, 80–81, 86
literal alexia, 79, 80–81, 86
occipital alexia, 79–80
parietal–temporal alexia, 80
phonological dyslexia, 151, 166, 190
posterior alexia, 79–80
pure alexia, 84, 151, 166, 168
surface dyslexia, 166, 190
verbal alexia, 79
Anomia, 153, 169–175
 category-specific anomia, 153
 concreteness, 169
 context, 172–173
 cueing and, 173–175
 exposure time, 172
 frequency, word, 169, 170–171
 grammatical category, 169
 length, word, 171
 markedness, 170
 modality specific anomia, 153
 motor anomia, 152
 nonaphasic anomias, 154
 operativity, 169
 paraphasic, 152
 prototypicality, 169–170
 pronounceability, 171
 psychogenic anomia, 154
 semantic anomia, 153
 semantic category, 169
 stimulus characteristics, 171
 stimulus uncertainity, 169
 treatment, 149, 168–175, 194–197
 word production anomia, 152–153
 word selection anomia, 153
Anomic aphasia, 173, 248, 249
 auditory comprehension, 43
 oral formulation, 155

305

Discourse (see also *Oral expression*) 10
  definition, 155
  expository, 157
  narrative, 156
  procedural, 156
  treatment, 181–184, 204–205
Discrimination
  auditory, 35–36, 37, 39–42, 51–55
  visual, 77–78, 81–87, 99–108

Efficacy, aphasia treatment,
    1–5, 150, 243, 252–258
Etiology
  of aphasia, 2–3, 245–247, 249, 250
  cerebrovascular accident, 2, 244,
    245–247, 249
  treatment results and, 2–3, 3–4, 253
Evaluation (see also *Tests*), 12
  aphasia tests, 5, 34, 42, 44, 127
    180, 246, 247
  testing schedule, 247, 250
Expression. See *Graphic
    expression; Oral expression*

Feedback, 23

Gestural and gestural-verbal
    communication, 127–140
  American Sign Language (ASL),
    78, 88, 131
  Amer-Ind, 78, 88, 130–131
  classification, 131–132
  decoding problems, 88–89,
    111–114
  definition, description, 129
  gesticulation, 87, 129, 133
  hemiplegia and, 134
  iconic gestures, 78, 89, 130, 131
  indicative gestures, 88
  mimicry, 87
  noniconic gestures, 131
  nonreferential gestures, 133
  pantomime, 87, 88
  propositional versus
    nonpropositional gestures,
    131–132, 135
  referential gestures, 133
  representational versus
    nonrepresentational gestures, 132
  response to treatment, 129–131
  simple versus complex gestures, 132
  speech acts, 136–140, 144–146
  static versus dynamic gestures,

129, 130, 132
  subpropositional gestures, 88
  symbolic gestures, 87–88, 89, 132
  treatment activities, 111–114,
    141, 146
  treatment guidelines and areas,
    10, 87–89, 132–140
Gestures. See *Gestural and gestural-
    verbal communication*
Global aphasia, 248, 249
  evolution of treatment, 4
  gestural recognition, 88
  oral formulation, 155
  reading, oral, 167
  recognition of spelling, 90
  recovery, 255, 256
  treatment profile, 268–269, 270, 272
  Visual Action Therapy, 214–215,
    216
  visual recognition of categories, 85
Grammatical form class, 44, 92, 162,
    167, 175
  adjective, 44, 166, 172, 176, 220,
    221, 225
  noun, 44, 67, 92, 166, 167, 169, 172,
    176, 177, 212, 220, 221, 225
  particle, 167, 177
  preposition, 93, 172, 177, 225
  pronoun, 44, 183
  verb, 44, 92, 166, 169, 177, 212,
    220, 221, 225
Graphic expression (see also
    Agraphia), 208–211, 221–241
  classifying deficits, 208–209
  motor problems, 209–211
  naming, factors affecting, 211–223
  physical letter code problems,
    210–211
  recovery, 23–24, 258, 259
  sentence formulation, factors
    affecting, 223–227
  treatment activities, 229–241
  treatment guidelines and areas, 10,
    214–228
Group therapy, 2
  individual therapy versus, 4

Hearing criteria, 246, 247
Hemiplegia
  Broca's aphasia and, 81, 152
  gestures and, 130, 134
  severity, 250, 251
  writing and, 209–210

–NOTES–

-NOTES-

-NOTES-

-NOTES-

–NOTES–

–NOTES–